Farzeen Firoozi
Editor

Interpretation of Basic and Advanced Urodynamics

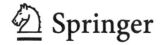

Editor
Farzeen Firoozi, MD FACS
Hofstra Northwell School of Medicine
Director, FPMRS
Associate Professor of Urology
The Smith Institute for Urology
Lake Success, NY, USA

ISBN 978-3-319-43245-8   ISBN 978-3-319-43247-2 (eBook)
DOI 10.1007/978-3-319-43247-2

Library of Congress Control Number: 2016958613

© Springer International Publishing Switzerland 2017
This work is subject to copyright. All rights are reserved by the Publisher, whether the whole or part of the material is concerned, specifically the rights of translation, reprinting, reuse of illustrations, recitation, broadcasting, reproduction on microfilms or in any other physical way, and transmission or information storage and retrieval, electronic adaptation, computer software, or by similar or dissimilar methodology now known or hereafter developed.
The use of general descriptive names, registered names, trademarks, service marks, etc. in this publication does not imply, even in the absence of a specific statement, that such names are exempt from the relevant protective laws and regulations and therefore free for general use.
The publisher, the authors and the editors are safe to assume that the advice and information in this book are believed to be true and accurate at the date of publication. Neither the publisher nor the authors or the editors give a warranty, express or implied, with respect to the material contained herein or for any errors or omissions that may have been made.

Printed on acid-free paper

This Springer imprint is published by Springer Nature
The registered company is Springer International Publishing AG
The registered company address is: Gewerbestrasse 11, 6330 Cham, Switzerland

*To my wife Kelly
and my sons Sam, Alex, and Jack*

Foreword

Despite the impressive advances in the management of lower urinary tract disorders in the last two decades, the single most important method of evaluating the lower urinary tract remains urodynamic testing. A complete and nuanced understanding of all aspects of urodynamics—from equipment set-up, to troubleshooting and interpretation of findings—is critical for understanding lower urinary tract pathology. Without such an understanding, the clinician cannot adequately assess and manage many of the patients seen in a typical FPMRS or general urology clinic. Education in this regard cannot be underestimated.

This text, *Interpretation of Basic and Advanced Urodynamics*, fills a critical role, enabling clinicians to understand the entire field of urodynamics. Edited by Dr. Farzeen Firoozi, an accomplished FPMRS surgeon based at The Smith Institute for Urology, Hofstra Northwell Health School of Medicine, this text explores urodynamics through the paradigm of specific disorders. Each chapter describes a particular condition, and the role and utility of urodynamics within that specific condition is described. Chapters cover topics ranging from Female Stress Incontinence to the Augmented Lower Urinary Tract to Pelvic Organ Prolapse. Thus, the learner can appreciate the applicability and interpretation of urodynamic studies in the context of these specific complaints/disorders.

Dr. Firoozi has assembled a cast of internationally renowned authors who are eminently qualified to review these topics. Furthermore, the chapters contain clinical vignettes to exemplify the conditions described and in a sense add experiential learning to these subjects as opposed to learning from just dry text. I have no doubt that this book will serve as an important guide to urologists, gynecologists, and others who deal with patients with lower urinary tract disorders and facilitate accurate diagnosis and treatment for their patients.

Cleveland, OH, USA   Howard B. Goldman

Preface

Urodynamic studies have been an essential tool of voiding dysfunction specialists for many decades. They provide the information needed to define the function—or dysfunction as it were—of patients who suffer from a variety of lower urinary tract issues. Additionally, they bring into the fold an understanding of the anatomy of the lower urinary tract. Although it is a well-established diagnostic study, there is no universally accepted method of interpretation for urodynamic studies, despite attempts made by many governing bodies and societies in the field of female pelvic medicine and reconstructive surgery.

Interpretation of Basic and Advanced Urodynamics was borne out of the desire to create an atlas of tracings that covers all categories of voiding dysfunction. Most previous textbooks on the subject of urodynamics have been mainly instructive with respect to carrying out these studies. The goal of this book has been to present real clinical cases and the urodynamics used to evaluate and treat these patients. Careful thought has been put into choosing these cases as they reflect every common as well as uncommon disease state that can affect voiding function. In addition to the initial chapter reviewing the basics of setting up, trouble shooting, and standardization of interpretation, the urodynamic tracings in subsequent chapters along with their interpretations have been provided by experts in the field.

The hope is that this atlas of urodynamics will serve as a reference for urologists and gynecologists, to be used as a urodynamic benchmark.

New York, NY   Farzeen Firoozi

Contents

1. **Equipment, Setup, and Troubleshooting for Basic and Advanced Urodynamics** 1
   Karyn S. Eilber, Tom Feng, and Jennifer Tash Anger

2. **Terminology/Standard Interpretative Format for Basic and Advanced Urodynamics** 9
   Drew A. Freilich and Eric S. Rovner

3. **Overactive Bladder: Non-neurogenic** 21
   Marisa M. Clifton and Howard B. Goldman

4. **Overactive Bladder: Neurogenic** 27
   Alana M. Murphy and Patrick J. Shenot

5. **Female Stress Urinary Incontinence** 35
   Nitin Sharma, Farzeen Firoozi, and Elizabeth Kavaler

6. **Male Stress Urinary Incontinence** 43
   Ricardo Palmerola and Farzeen Firoozi

7. **Bladder Outlet Obstruction: Male Non-neurogenic** 55
   Christopher Hartman and David Y. Chan

8. **Bladder Outlet Obstruction: Female Non-neurogenic** 65
   William D. Ulmer and Elise J.B. De

9. **Neurogenic Bladder Obstruction** 79
   Seth A. Cohen and Shlomo Raz

10. **Iatrogenic Female Bladder Outlet Obstruction** 89
    Sandip Vasavada

11. **Pelvic Organ Prolapse** 93
    Courtenay K. Moore

12. **Augmented Lower Urinary Tract** 101
    Shilo Rosenberg and David A. Ginsberg

13. **Adolescent/Early Adult Former Pediatric Neurogenic Patients: Special Considerations** 109
    Benjamin Abelson and Hadley M. Wood

14. **Lower Urinary Tract Anomalies** 125
    Michael Ingber

Index 133

Contributors

Benjamin Abelson, M.D. Glickman Urological and Kidney Institute, Department of Urology, Cleveland Clinic, Cleveland, OH, USA

Jennifer Tash Anger, M.D., M.P.H. Department of Surgery, Division of Urology, Cedars-Sinai Medical Center, Beverly Hills, CA, USA

David Y. Chan, M.D. Department of Urology, Hofstra North Shore—LIJ, The Smith Institute for Urology, New Hyde Park, NY, USA

Marisa M. Clifton, M.D. Department of Urology, Cleveland Clinic Foundation, Cleveland, OH, USA

Seth A. Cohen, M.D. Division of Urology and Urologic Oncology, Department of Surgery, Glendora, CA, USA

Elise J.B. De, M.D. Department of Surgery, Division of Urology, Albany Medical Center, Albany, NY, USA

Karyn S. Eilberg, M.D. Department of Surgery, Division of Urology, Cedars-Sinai Medical Center, Beverly Hills, CA, USA

Tom Feng, M.D. Department of Surgery, Division of Urology, Cedars Sinai Medical Center, Los Angeles, CA, USA

Farzeen Firoozi, M.D., F.A.C.S. Department of Urology, Northwell Health System, Center for Advanced Medicine, The Arthur Smith Institute of Urology, New Hyde Park, NY, USA

Drew A. Freilich, M.D. Department of Urology, Medical University of South Carolina, Charleston, SC, USA

David A. Ginsberg, M.D. Department of Urology, Keck School of Medicine at USC, Los Angeles, CA, USA

Howard B. Goldman, M.D. Department of Urology, Cleveland Clinic Foundation, Cleveland, OH, USA

Christopher Hartman, M.D. Department of Urology, Hofstra North Shore—LIJ, The Smith Institute for Urology, New Hyde Park, NY, USA

Michael Ingber, M.D. Department of Urology, Atlantic Health System, Denville, NJ, USA

Elizabeth Kavaler, M.D. Department of Urology, New York Presbyterian Hospital, New York, NY, USA

Courtenay K. Moore, M.D. Glickman Urological Institute, Cleveland Clinic, Cleveland, OH, USA

Alana M. Murphy, M.D. Department of Urology, Thomas Jefferson University Hospital, Philadelphia, PA, USA

Ricardo Palmerola, M.D., M.S. Department of Urology, Northwell Health System, Center for Advanced Medicine, The Arthur Smith Institute for Urology, New Hyde Park, NY, USA

Shlomo Raz, M.D. Division of Pelvic Medicine and Reconstructive Surgery, Department of Urology, UCLA, Los Angeles, CA, USA

Shilo Rosenberg, M.D. Department of Urology, Keck School of Medicine at USC, Los Angeles, CA, USA

Eric S. Rovner, M.D. Department of Urology, Medical University of South Carolina, Charleston, SC, USA

Nitin Sharma, M.D. Department of Urology, Lenox Hill Hospital, New York, NY, USA

Patrick J. Shenot, M.D. Department of Urology, Thomas Jefferson University Hospital, Philadelphia, PA, USA

William D. Ulmer, M.D. Department of Surgery, Division of Urology, Albany Medical Center, Albany, NY, USA

Sandip Vasavada, M.D. Department of Urology, Cleveland Clinic, Cleveland, OH, USA

Hadley M. Wood, M.D., F.A.C.S. Glickman Urological and Kidney Institute, Department of Urology, Cleveland Clinic, Cleveland, OH, USA

Equipment, Setup, and Troubleshooting for Basic and Advanced Urodynamics

Karyn S. Eilber, Tom Feng, and Jennifer Tash Anger

1.1 Introduction

Urodynamics (UDS) refers to a set of diagnostic tests that allows the clinician to accurately assess the function of the lower urinary tract. By measuring pressure and flow, UDS provides information regarding the functional pathophysiology of a patient's symptoms. The American Urological Association clinical practice guidelines regarding the indications for urodynamics broadly describe two categories of patients who may benefit from UDS: (1) patients in whom an accurate diagnosis is needed to direct treatment and the diagnosis cannot be determined by history, physical examination, and basic tests alone and (2) patients whose lower urinary tract disease can cause upper urinary tract deterioration if not diagnosed and treated [1].

Interest in the dynamics of micturition has existed for centuries; however, the term *urodynamics* is attributed to David M. Davis [2]. One of the earliest UDS prototypes was developed by von Garrelts, who employed the simultaneous use of a pressure transducer and measurement of voided urine volume as a function of time [3, 4]. Soon after this, the principles of urethral closure pressure and EMG were described [4]. Since that time, UDS equipment has become more sophisticated and "user-friendly" such that practitioners perform both simple (single-channel) and complex (multi-channel) urodynamics in the office. The primary goal of this chapter is to provide the clinician with a framework to create a urodynamics laboratory in the office setting including equipment options, setup, and troubleshooting.

1.2 Equipment

1.2.1 Simple Versus Complex UDS Systems

A simple urodynamics study consists of a cystometrogram (CMG) combined with uroflowmetry. The addition of intra abdominal and/or intraurethral pressure measurements and pelvic floor electromyography converts simple UDS to complex, or multi-channel, UDS. The clinician should keep in mind that while multi-channel UDS machines are able to perform both simple and complex UDS, a single-channel UDS machine is not capable of measuring more than intravesical pressure. Hence, the ability of a multi-channel UDS machine to measure both intravesical and intraabdominal pressures provides the most accurate assessment of lower urinary tract function.

1.2.1.1 Simple UDS Systems

A simple urodynamics system is an appropriate choice for the clinician who desires only basic information regarding lower urinary tract function. This system usually only reports intravesical pressure and uroflowmetry. An important consideration for the clinician is that the intravesical pressure measured by simple UDS may not reflect the true clinical scenario. Without measurement of intraabdominal pressure, simple UDS cannot differentiate between an increase in intravesical pressure generated by the detrusor muscle versus an increase in the surrounding intraabdominal pressure.

While more complicated clinical scenarios may not be accurately assessed by simple UDS, a single-channel UDS system does have its advantages. Generally, a simple UDS machine is less expensive than a multi-channel machine. The cost of a simple UDS machine ranges from $10,000 to $15,000, compared to complex UDS systems which may

K.S. Eilber, M.D. (✉) • J.T. Anger, M.D., M.P.H.
Department of Surgery, Division of Urology, Cedars-Sinai Medical Center, 99 North La Cienega Boulevard, Suite 307, Beverly Hills, CA 90211, USA
e-mail: karyn.eilber@cshs.org; Jennifer.anger@cshs.org

T. Feng, M.D.
Department of Surgery, Division of Urology, Cedars Sinai Medical Center, 8635 W Third Street, Suite 1070 West, Los Angeles, CA 90048, USA
e-mail: tom.feng@cshs.org

cost as much as $80,000 (USD). Furthermore, as the name implies, the equipment and setup required to perform simple urodynamics are much less complicated than a multi-channel system. The basic requirements, in addition to the actual urodynamics machine, are a urethral catheter to measure bladder pressure and a uroflowmeter.

1.2.1.2 Complex UDS Systems

The main differences between simple and complex UDS are the addition of an intraabdominal catheter and electromyography as well as a computer that can report multiple measurements: intravesical pressure (P_{ves}), intraabdominal pressure (P_{abd}), urethral pressure profile (UPP), electromyography (EMG), uroflowmetry (UF), volume instilled into the bladder, and volume voided. For the purposes of this textbook, the remainder of this chapter will focus on complex (multi-channel) UDS.

Intravesical Catheters

When choosing the type of intravesical catheter for UDS, performance of simple versus complex UDS, patient anatomy, machine requirements, and cost all need to be considered. Both simple and complex UDS typically use dual-lumen, fluid-filled urethral catheters to measure intravesical pressure. One lumen of the catheter functions as a channel to fill the bladder, while the other lumen is connected to an external pressure sensor (transducer). Urethral catheters with a third lumen are also available that can measure UPP. Connection tubing is used to attach the intravesical catheter to the transducer, which then converts pressure into electrical energy that appears as a tracing on a computer screen [5].

Catheters from different manufacturers are generally compatible with multiple UDS systems. The majority of UDS are performed with fluid-filled catheters, but other options include air-charged and electronic (micro tip) catheters. The International Continence Society (ICS) recommends the use of fluid-filled urethral catheters and tubing for increased accuracy [6].

The size of urethral catheters ranges from 4 to 10 French (Fr). UDS catheters are also available with a curved (Coudé) tip. Coudé tip catheters are especially useful for male patients as UDS catheters are smaller and more pliable than most urethral catheters such that the curved tip is often necessary to negotiate the curve of the male urethra. In addition, a large proportion of men undergoing UDS have benign prostatic hyperplasia and further benefit from the use of a Coudé tip catheter.

Finally, cost may also influence the choice of catheter. Careful consideration should be given to the cost of catheters, especially if catheters from different manufacturers are not compatible with a specific urodynamics machine. As the catheters are disposable, cost differences can be significant over time.

Intraabdominal Catheters

The intravesical pressure is influenced by abdominal pressure; thus, measuring P_{ves} alone is not the most reliable method of determining bladder function. Detrusor pressure (P_{det}) is a calculated value and is the difference between the measured intravesical pressure and the intraabdominal pressure (Fig. 1.1).

$$P_{det} = P_{ves} - P_{abd}$$

As simple UDS systems only measure intravesical pressure, P_{det} can only be determined when the intraabdominal pressure is measured during multi-channel urodynamics. The ICS recommends a rectal balloon catheter be used to measure P_{abd}, and this recommendation is followed by most practitioners [6, 7]. Nonetheless, the vagina is an acceptable option for female patients who prefer not to have a rectal catheter and is commonly used in urogynecologic practices with the caveat that this method is not as accurate and prone to artifacts, especially in women with pelvic organ prolapse [8, 9]. In cases where the rectum is absent, P_{abd} can be measured by placing the catheter in an intestinal stoma. Regardless of where the intraabdominal catheter is placed, the catheter design is dual lumen with one lumen to assess pressure and the other lumen to fill a balloon at the end of the catheter. The balloon is usually 5 milliliters (mL) and catheter size ranges from 8 to 12 Fr. The ICS recommends the use of water-based transducers to measure both intravesical and intraabdominal pressure [6].

Fluid Media

Sterile water or saline are commonly used fluid media to fill the bladder during an urodynamics study. It may be cost effective to use 500 mL bags of fluid as functional bladder capacity usually does not exceed this volume. When assessing for incontinence without fluoroscopy, it can be useful to add indigo carmine or methylene blue to the fluid so that leakage can be readily identified during the study. If fluoroscopy is used for video-urodynamics, it is necessary to use radiographic contrast as the fluid media.

Electrodes

During voiding, intraurethral pressure decreases prior to the detrusor contracting and this, in turn, is related to pelvic floor relaxation [4]. Franksson and Peterson are credited with EMG studies of the pelvic floor and form the basis for incorporation of EMG into UDS tests [10]. EMG is particularly useful in the diagnosis of functional obstruction and can be performed with surface, needle, intravaginal, or rectal electrodes. Widespread use of surface EMG is likely driven by technical ease and patient comfort. Examples of intravesical and intraabdominal catheters and surface EMG electrodes are shown in Fig. 1.2.

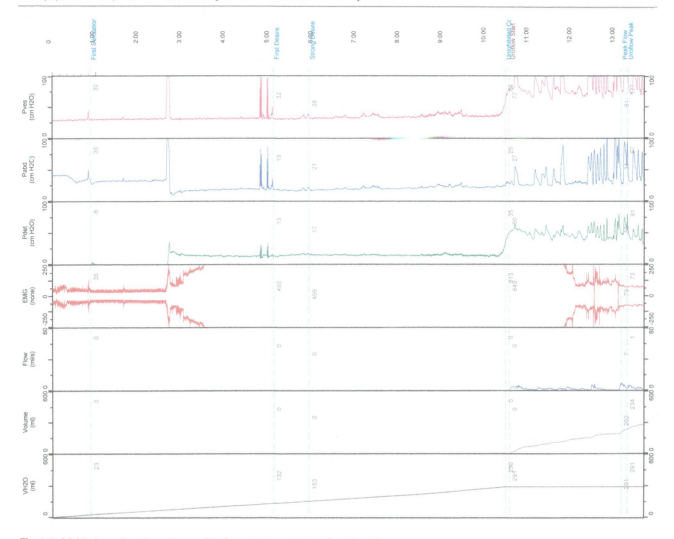

Fig. 1.1 Multi-channel urodynamics graphical report demonstrating $P_{det} = P_{ves} - P_{abd}$

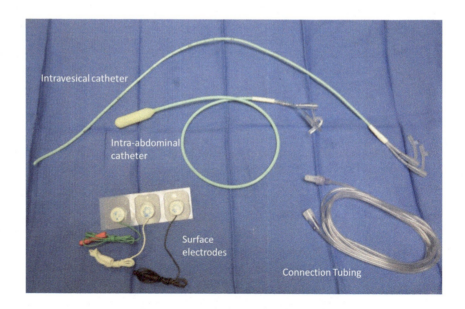

Fig. 1.2 Intravesical catheter, intra-abdominal catheter, connection tubing, and EMG electrodes

Uroflow Meter

Uroflowmetry is the measurement of the rate of flow of urine over time, typically reported in milliliters per second [1]. As the essence of UDS is the ability to determine the relationship between bladder pressure and urine flow rate, most UDS systems include a uroflowmetry device although a graduated beaker to collect urine and a uroflow meter stand are usually not included with the UDS system.

It is often overlooked that the uroflow meter purchased with a UDS system can be used alone when only uroflowmetry is desired. This can potentially result in cost and space savings by obviating the need for both a urodynamics machine and a separate uroflow meter.

Exam Table

A multi-positional exam table controlled by a foot pedal is the most advantageous as it allows the patient to be seamlessly repositioned during the study from the supine or lithotomy position for catheter placement to a seated position for the study.

When video-UDS is being performed, a radiolucent exam table or commode chair must be used if the study is performed supine or in the sitting position, respectively. An alternative to using a radiolucent exam table or commode is performing the study in a standing position.

Wireless Systems

In recent years, wireless UDS systems have become available such that information obtained from the pressure transducers and uroflow meter is wirelessly transmitted to the computer. Values for intravesical and intraabdominal pressure, volume infused, uroflowmetry, volume voided, and UPP are uploaded without a direct connection to the computer. The most obvious advantage of a wireless system is having fewer cables. In addition, these systems also have a smaller footprint and provide greater flexibility in terms of equipment setup, as computer proximity to the UDS machine is not dictated by cable length.

Software

Available software that is compatible with certain UDS systems is an important consideration when purchasing equipment. Some of the software options are graphical appearance of the study, layout options for reporting patient history and study data, nomograms, and computerized interpretation of the study. When acquiring a UDS machine, options and cost for software upgrades should also be considered.

Printing Data Versus Transmission to EMR

Once UDS data are acquired, the computer hard drive is able to store the results, but most clinicians also want the data in each patient's medical record. Options of data transfer to a patient's medical record are either (1) print a hard copy of the study to either place in a patient's paper chart or scan into an electronic chart or (2) have the electronic data directly sent into the patient's electronic medical record (EMR).

Table 1.1 Software available for data collection

UDS manufacturer	Software
Laborie (Mississauga, Ontario, Canada)	i-List®, UroConsole®
Andromeda (Taufkirchen/Potzham, Germany)	AUDACT®
Prometheus (Dover, New Hampshire, USA)	Morpheus®

When acquiring a UDS system, a printer is often included. If not, the compatibility of a printer with the UDS system must be determined. With multichannel UDS, each channel may be assigned a different color for ease of interpretation; however, the cost of color ink is an additional consideration.

For clinicians who have an existing EMR, compatibility of UDS software must also be considered, as there are significant advantages of direct data transfer. Both time and cost of printing a report are avoided, and the UDS data can be stored both in the UDS system hard drive as well as in the EMR. Engineers from both the UDS equipment manufacturer as well as the EMR vendor are usually necessary to establish a direct link between the UDS machine and the EMR. Examples of software currently available are listed in Table 1.1.

Fluoroscopy

Video-urodynamics is the addition of a voiding cystourethrogram to the pressure-flow study. The most commonly applied imaging is fluoroscopy. In the past fluoroscopy units were often large and extremely expensive, but modern units are mobile and with a relatively small footprint such that video-UDS can be performed in the office. The cost of a fluoroscopy unit may be offset by using it for purposes other than video-UDS. In addition to video-UDS, the authors use their fluoroscopy unit for cystograms, retrograde urethrograms, evaluation of stones or stent position, nephrostograms, and percutaneous sacral nerve evaluation trials.

Safety requirements for fluoroscopy vary by region, but items to consider include physician fluoroscopy licensing (and any other medical personnel who will be operating the fluoroscopy machine), state registration of the fluoroscopy machine, evaluation of the machine by a radiation physicist, lead lining of the examination room, and protective shielding for the clinician and patient. The radiology licenses also need to be posted in the room where the imaging will be performed. Furthermore, radiation badges must be maintained and submitted for regular monitoring.

Purchase and Maintenance

Purchasing a UDS system is a significant investment, and the buyer must choose whether to purchase a system or lease a system. The latter may also include an option to purchase the equipment at the end of the lease. If available, a refurbished system can be a consideration to minimize cost. Regardless of whether new or refurbished equipment is obtained, some type of service agreement is advantageous. On multiple occasions the authors have had to troubleshoot the system online with the manufacturer, which is included in our urodynamics machine's service agreement. Without such a service agreement, the issue may not have been resolved in real time, and/or the cost of each encounter would have been significant.

1.3 Setup

1.3.1 Equipment Setup

The size of the examination room where the UDS study will be performed is determined by whether simple or complex UDS is being performed. Often simple UDS can be performed in a regular examination room, whereas an examination room that can accommodate an adjustable examination table, computer, and urodynamics tower is needed for complex UDS. Additional space is necessary if fluoroscopy will be used for video-UDS. The room should be Wi-Fi enabled or have Ethernet capability in the event that remote electronic repairs need to be made and for transmission of data to an EMR. The examination table should be positioned in relation to the entryway as to maintain privacy and wheelchair accessibility. With increasing use of wireless UDS systems, the computer location is no longer dictated by cable location (Fig. 1.3).

It is strongly recommended that a qualified service technician employed by the UDS machine manufacturer assist in the initial equipment setup and be readily available when the first UDS tests are performed. The technician is also invaluable with instillation and customization of software programs. One area of customization is the order of the urodynamic values that are displayed on the computer screen, and this is dictated by clinician preference. Also customizable are rates of bladder filling and the format of data reporting. Some software programs are able to generate a document that includes both patient history and a written description of the urodynamic findings.

If video-UDS are to be performed, a radiation physicist should be consulted and a county inspector usually needs to evaluate the fluoroscopy machine. Many institutions require that a medical equipment engineer also inspect the equipment before use.

1.3.2 Supplies

A properly and consistently arranged supply table or procedure tray and a readily available assistant make the most efficient use of time and reduce waste. The UDS computer should already be turned on with the appropriate program open and the patient information entered prior to the patient entering the exam room. The catheters, connecting tubing, fluid media, electrodes, sterile gloves, lubricant, and skin cleanser should all be on a table or tray close to the patient (Fig. 1.3). When a patient has significant vaginal prolapse that needs reduction, either a pessary or vaginal packing should also be readily accessible. The assistant must be able to immediately pass all supplies to the clinician and maintain sterility when necessary.

Fig. 1.3 Video-urodynamics setup

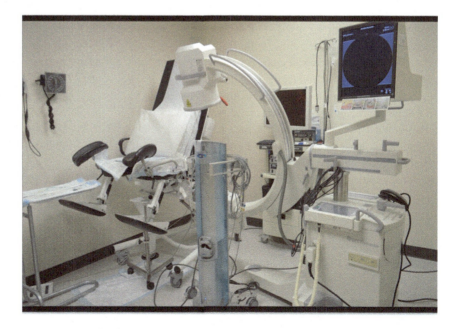

1.3.3 Patient Preparation

Although patients understand the necessity and value of UDS, the clinician must respect the patient's choice to be subjected to invasive testing. The authors routinely provide written information to patients at the time of test scheduling that includes reasons for performing the test, what the test entails, how long to expect to be at the office, and medical conditions that may require antibiotic prophylaxis. The authors follow AUA guidelines regarding antibiotic prophylaxis for urodynamic studies, which recommends antimicrobial prophylaxis only for patients with certain risk factors: advanced age, anatomic abnormalities of the urinary tract, malnutrition, smoking, chronic steroid use, immunodeficiency, indwelling catheters, bacterial colonization, coexistent infection, and prolonged hospitalization [11, 12].

If a woman is of reproductive age, confirmation that the patient is not pregnant must be determined before performing fluoroscopy.

1.3.4 Patient Setup

Both male and female patients should be in low lithotomy position for urethral and rectal catheter placement. The great majority of women tolerate urethral placement without topical anesthesia; however, if a female patient has significant discomfort at baseline, then topical anesthesia is used. Topical anesthesia is applied for most male patients unless they perform self-catheterization.

To maintain sterility and avoid changing examination gloves, the urethral catheter is placed first using standard sterile technique. Without changing gloves, the EMG surface electrodes followed by the rectal catheter are placed. A cystoscope should be readily available in the event that the urethral catheter cannot be inserted. The catheters should be secured to the patient's leg either with adhesive tape or some type of catheter securing device. For female patients, the authors secure the urethral catheter to the inner thigh at the level of the urethra. For male patients, the glans needs to be free of any lubricant used to insert the catheter, and a strip of adhesive tape is placed starting at the proximal glans and extending at least 2 cm onto the urethral catheter itself. A second piece of tape is placed circumferentially around the glans to hold the first strip in place. It is important that any personnel who insert catheters possess appropriate medical licensure.

Once the catheters are placed, the patient is changed to a seated position. The authors maintain a seated position for female patients as this is the position in which most women void. If the examination table does not allow testing in the seated position, the patient can be changed to a standing position, and a urine collection device designed to be placed between a woman's legs to collect urine and funnel it into a uroflow meter can be used. Male patients are usually studied in the standing position unless the patient indicates that he voids in the seated position. Patients who cannot stand or maintain a seated position, such as quadriplegic patients, must have the test performed while supine.

Following catheter placement, the urethral and rectal catheters are connected to the external transducer via connection tubing. When the test is completed, all catheters, connection tubing, and EMG electrodes are discarded.

1.3.5 Establishing Zero Pressure

The ICS recommends that "zero pressure is the surrounding atmospheric pressure" [6]. Furthermore, the ICS has established reference height as the upper edge of the symphysis pubis [6]. In order to establish zero pressure as the surrounding atmospheric pressure, the transducer must be "open" to the environment and "closed" to the patient. This can be achieved using a three-way stopcock. A fluid-filled syringe is attached to one tap, the tap attached to the patient is in the closed position, and the remaining tap is open to the environment. The fluid-filled syringe is used to flush out any air bubbles prior to setting zero. Once zero pressure has been established, the open tap is sealed with a cap (Fig. 1.4a–c).

1.4 Troubleshooting

1.4.1 Urodynamics Program Open but Unable to Perform Test

- Confirm that all necessary patient information and other required data have been entered.
- Confirm that any necessary Bluetooth and Wi-Fi connections are set appropriately and internet connection is established.

1.4.2 Urodynamics Program Running but No Pressure Readings

- Confirm catheters inserted far enough into appropriate lumen.
- Confirm all catheters securely connected to appropriate transducers.
- Confirm proper position of pressure transducer stopcock.
- Flush all connection tubing to eliminate any air bubbles.

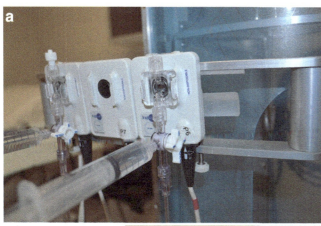
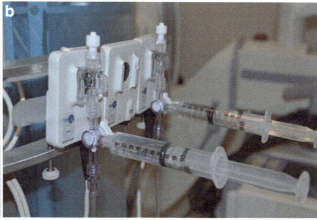
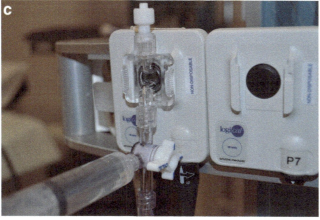

Fig. 1.4 (**a**) Three-way stopcock positioned so that system open to atmosphere. (**b, c**) Three-way stopcock positioned so that system closed to atmosphere

1.4.3 Pressures Detected but Intravesical Pressure Remains Low and Unchanged

- Urethral catheter tip may be in wall of bladder and will correct itself as bladder fills.
- Urethral catheter tip may be in a bladder diverticulum so repositioning catheter will result in normal pressure fluctuations.
- Urethral catheter inadvertently placed in vaginal canal.

1.4.4 Urethral or Rectal Pressure Suddenly Drops

- Confirm that urethral or rectal catheter still in bladder or rectum, respectively.
- Check for any kinks in catheter or connection tubing.

1.4.5 No Intraabdominal Pressure Recording

- Inflate rectal catheter balloon with more fluid.
- Remove impacted stool.

1.4.6 Unable to Advance Urethral Catheter into the Bladder

- Attempt to pass Coudé catheter if available.
- Insert urethral catheter into bladder under direct vision by passing catheter alongside a cystoscope.

1.4.7 Measured Volume of Fluid Medium Instilled Does Not Equal Starting Volume of Fluid Medium Used

- Check pump chamber functioning properly.
- Pump may need to be calibrated.

1.4.8 No Flow of Fluid Medium

- Check for any kinking or other obstruction of connection tubing.
- Flush connecting tubing to eliminate any air bubbles.

References

1. Winters JC, Dmochowski RR, Goldman HB, et al. Adult urodynamics: AUA/SUFU guideline. J Urol. 2012;188(6 Suppl):2464–72.
2. Davis DM. The hydrodynamics of the upper urinary tract (urodynamic). Ann Surg. 1954;140(6):839–49.
3. von Garrelts B. Micturition in the normal male. Acta Chir Scand. 1958;114:197–210.
4. Abrams P. Urodynamic techniques. In: Urodynamics. 3rd ed. London: Springer; 2006. p. 17.
5. Gray M. Traces: making sense of urodynamic testing. Urol Nurs. 2010;30(5):267–75.
6. Schafer W, Abrams P, Liao L, et al. Good urodynamic practices: uroflowmetry, filling cystometry, and pressure-flow studies. Neurourol Urodyn. 2002;21(3):261–74.
7. Gray M, Krissovich M. Characteristics of North American urodynamic centers: measuring lower urinary tract filling and storage function. Urol Nurs. 2004;24(1):30–8.
8. Dolan LM, Dixon WE, Brown K, et al. Randomized comparison of vaginal and rectal measurement of intra-abdominal pressure during subtracted dual-channel cystometry. Urology. 2005;65(6):1059–63.
9. Wall LL, Hewitt JK, Helms MJ. Are vaginal and rectal pressures equivalent approximations of one another for the purpose of performing subtracted cystometry? Obstet Gynecol. 1995;85(4):488–93.
10. Franksson C, Petersen I. Electromyographic investigation of disturbances in the striated muscle of the urethral sphincter. Br J Urol. 1955;27:154–61.
11. Wolf JS, Bennett CJ, Dmochowski RR, et al. Best practice policy statement on urologic surgery antimicrobial prophylaxis. J Urol. 2009;182(2):799–800.
12. Schaeffer AJ, Schaeffer EM. Infections of the urinary tract. In: Wein AJ, Kavoussi LR, Novick AC, et al., editors. Campbell-Walsh urology, vol. 1. 9th ed. Philadelphia: Saunders-Elsevier; 2007. p. 223–303.

Terminology/Standard Interpretative Format for Basic and Advanced Urodynamics

Drew A. Freilich and Eric S. Rovner

2.1 Introduction

Urodynamics (UDS) are the dynamic study of the transport, storage, and evacuation of urine [1]. UDS consists of a number of studies including uroflowmetry, post void residual measurement, filling and voiding cystometry, and sometimes urethral pressure measurement. Often fluoroscopy is used concurrently to evaluate the dynamic anatomy of urinary tract. These tests measure and assess various processes intrinsic and extrinsic to the lower urinary tract. UDS can assist in the diagnosis, prognosis, and treatment regimens. The term urodynamics was first coined by Dr. David Davis in 1954 [2]. Since then, there has been an exponential increase in the utilization of UDS by healthcare practitioners including urologists.

In more than 60 years since Dr. Davis' initial reports, there is now a broad base of literature, and there are many textbooks devoted to the performance and interpretation of urodynamics. Despite this there is no standardized methodology or guidelines that dictate the manner in which urodynamic tracings are interpreted.

The amount of information produced during a routine PFUD study can be imposing to fully comprehend, understand, and properly interpret. For a given study, the modern electronic multichannel pressure-flow urodynamic machine produces a large amount of data in a graphical display usually supplemented with other information. The format varies depending on the type of urodynamic equipment, the specific study, and the end-user customization. Nevertheless, in most instances, the various channels on the graph represent a set of continuous variables over time including vesical and abdominal pressure recordings, urine flow rate and volume, infused volume, and potentially other signals as well. An event summary, annotations, nomograms, and other features now commonly found on commercially available urodynamics equipment add to the tremendous set of data available from a routine pressure-flow urodynamic (PFUD) study. In the same manner in which radiologists interpret their imaging studies, it is crucial to be systematic and organized in approaching the PFUD tracing in order to properly and completely distill the optimal amount of information from the study. It is quite possible to overlook salient and relevant features of a PFUD tracing especially in those cases where there exists one single overwhelming abnormality. Like the astute radiologist, the expert urodynamicist will not be dissuaded from completely interpreting the study even in the setting of a distracting feature so that other, subtler findings can be noted as well. Such nuances can be crucial in formulating an accurate interpretation of the study and should not be overlooked. The 9 "Cs" of PFUD are a method of organizing and interpreting the PFUD study in a simple, reliable, and practical manner [3]. In doing so, this system minimizes the potential for "missing" an important and relevant finding on the tracing. This framework is easy to understand, remember, and applicable to all PFUD studies for virtually all lower urinary conditions.

The utility of UDS in predicting postoperative outcomes has been called into question recently [4–6]. Collectively, these articles have suggested that UDS may not be needed prior to performing a sling for pure stress urinary incontinence in the uncomplicated patient. Whether these conclusions are truly valid for all patients is quite controversial. This underscores the importance of demonstrating good quality in the performance of these studies as well as the standardizing the interpretation of these studies. Such measures should maximize the utility of data in order to determine which patients most benefit from UDS. This is especially important as UDS studies are invasive, expensive, and potentially morbid.

D.A. Freilich, M.D. • E.S. Rovner, M.D. (✉)
Department of Urology, Medical University of South Carolina, 96 Jonathan Lucas Street, CSB 644, Charleston, SC 29425, USA
e-mail: freilicd@musc.edu; rovnere@musc.edu

2.2 The "9 Cs" of Urodynamics

In the functional classification as popularized by Wein, the micturition cycle consists of two phases: (1) bladder filling/urinary storage and (2) bladder emptying [7]. All voiding dysfunctions therefore can be categorized as abnormalities of one or both of these phases. This classification system also provides a useful framework for organizing the 9 "Cs."

The 9 "Cs" represent the nine essential features of the PFUDs tracing that represent a minimum interpretive data set. Each of the features begins with the letter "C" (Table 2.1). In the filling phase, the "Cs" consist of contractions (involuntary), compliance, continence, capacity, and coarse sensation. In the emptying phase, contractility, complete emptying, coordination, and clinical obstruction are evaluated.

The "Cs" are not specific for all types of urinary dysfunction nor all urodynamic abnormalities. Nevertheless, by organizing and interpreting a study within this framework, it provides an organizing thread from which to formulate a diagnosis and begin to assemble a management plan.

Of course all PFUD tracings should be interpreted in the context of the patient's history, physical examination, and other relevant studies. Additionally, reproducing the patient's symptoms or at least noting whether this was achieved during the study is also important in order to properly interpret the tracing and any abnormalities seen. Notwithstanding these limitations, it remains that a systematic and organized approach to interpretation of the PFUD tracing is likely to yield the most useful and complete set of data and optimize clinical care and outcomes.

Simply reviewing a UDS tracing is not sufficient to generate an accurate interpretation. The filling and voiding phases of the study are dynamic processes that are influenced by patient understanding of testing instructions (i.e., waiting for permission to void) and artifact (i.e., movement of uroflow detector during the test). Therefore, it is important that the person interpreting the UDS tracing is involved with the actual UDS study as knowledge of the testing environment will help differentiate artifacts from true findings.

Table 2.1 The 9 "Cs" of urodynamics

Filling and storage
Coarse sensation
Compliance
Contractions (involuntary detrusor)
Continence
Cystometric capacity
Emptying
Contractility
Coordination
Complete emptying
Clinical obstruction

2.2.1 Filling and Storage

The filling phase starts with the initiation of instillation of saline or contrast of a video urodynamic study and ends with "permission to void." Prior to giving permission to void, the provider performing the UDS needs to ensure that all questions regarding the filling and storage phase have been addressed. Once permission to void has been given, the emptying phase begins. It is helpful to have a recent voiding diary available prior to the UDS. The voiding diary will help assess how the UDS tracing reflects their voided volumes in a non-clinical environment (i.e., voided volumes or to estimate storage volumes which may affect filling rate).

2.2.1.1 Coarse Sensation

It is important to begin the study with an empty bladder. Thus, most often patients are catheterized prior to the start of the study. This will help ensure that the infused volumes at which sensations are recorded are accurate. It is also important to ensure that the recorded infused amount accurately reflects the actual infused amount. Such calibrations should be done regularly and periodically as routine maintenance of the urodynamic equipment. Bladder course sensation can be delayed in patients with poorly controlled diabetes and HIV. Sensation can be absent in patients with spinal cord injuries.

Patients should be informed of the study objectives prior to beginning testing and this is especially relevant when assessing sensation. They should be prompted to inform the person performing the study of:

1. First sensation of bladder filling (during filling cystometry, the sensation when he/she first becomes aware of bladder filling)
2. First desire to void (the feeling, during filling cystometry, that the patient would desire to pass urine and the next convenient moment, but voiding can be delayed if necessary)
3. Strong desire to void (during filling cystometry, as a persistent desire to void without the fear of leakage)
4. Maximum cystometric capacity (in patients with normal sensation, this is the volume at which the patient feels he/she can no longer delay micturition (has a strong desire to void))
5. Urgency (during filling cystometry, the sudden compelling desire to void at any time during the UDS) [1] (Fig. 2.1)

Filling sensation is very subjective and as such there is not a universally accepted normative value hence the term "coarse sensation" is utilized. Typical ranges are first sensation ~170–200 mL, first desire to void ~250 mL, strong desire to void ~400 mL, and maximum capacity ~480 mL

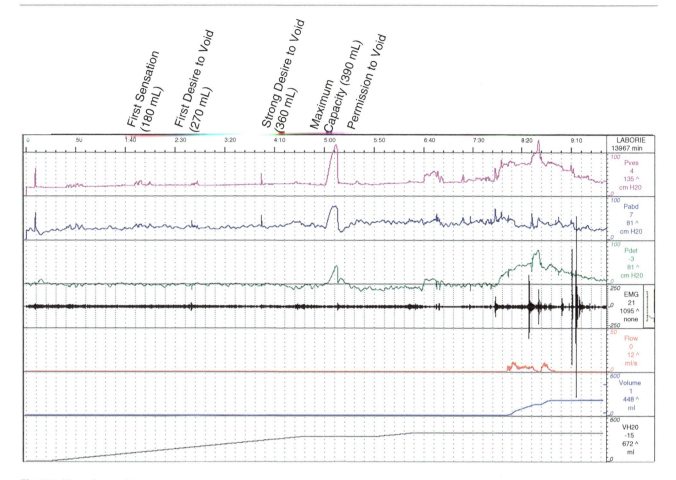

Fig. 2.1 Normal sensation

[8]. Reviewing a recent voiding diary may be helpful. Sensation is affected by the placement of a catheter in the bladder which may cause irritation and/or pain which may be erroneously interpreted as a sensation to void. Cold or overly warmed or too rapidly infused fluid can also affect bladder sensation. When documenting the interpretation of the UDS, tracing coarse sensation is usually reported as absent, reduced, or increased [9].

2.2.1.2 Compliance

Compliance reflects the passive viscoelastic properties of the bladder and is defined as the relationship between change in bladder volume and change in detrusor pressure [1]. Compliance is calculated by dividing the volume change of the bladder just prior to volitional micturition or the first involuntary bladder contraction by the detrusor pressure at that same point [1]. In a normally compliant bladder and in the absence of detrusor overactivity, the detrusor pressure should remain essentially unchanged during filling. Decreased bladder compliance is generally acknowledged as a risk factor for upper tract deterioration.

Despite the importance of this data point, there exists no universally accepted normative value. Compliance of less than 20 mL/cm H_2O is commonly used as the threshold below which is considered abnormal [10]. Occasionally, a prolonged involuntary bladder contraction (detrusor overactivity or DO) can be confused with true abnormal compliance. One way to differentiate between these is to stop infusing fluid and observe for a few minutes. Typically, pressures will return to baseline after a few minutes with DO, whereas pressures will remain high in abnormal compliance. Video urodynamics/VCUG can be helpful as high-grade reflux and large bladder diverticulum can act as a "pop-off" masking underlying abnormal compliance.

Testing of the detrusor leak point pressure (DLPP) in patients with abnormal compliance can be helpful in risk assessment of future upper tract deterioration. DLPP is defined as "lowest value of the detrusor pressure at which leakage is observed in the absence of abdominal strain or detrusor contraction" [11]. A DLPP of greater than 40 is considered deleterious to the upper tracts [12]. However, in certain individuals, a DLPP of less than 40 may also put the upper tracts at risk (Fig. 2.2).

Pelvic radiation, denervation from radical pelvic surgery, neurogenic bladder, and indwelling Foley are common etiologies of abnormal bladder compliance. Patients who have

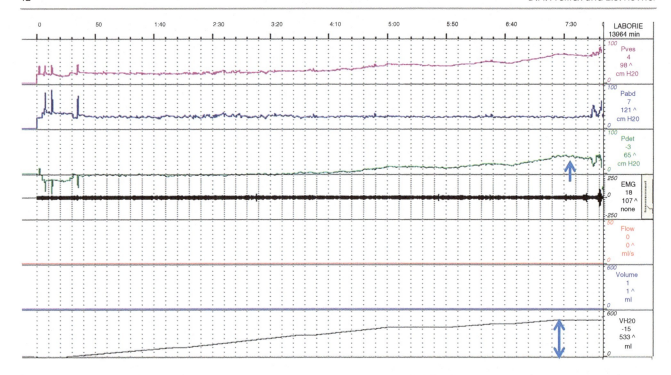

Fig. 2.2 Decreased compliance. The *single arrow* denotes a change in pressure of 41 cm H$_2$O. The *double arrow* demonstrates a change in volume of 493 mL. Compliance = (ΔVolume/ΔP_{det}) = 493 mL/41 cm = 12 mL/cm H$_2$O

abnormal compliance with a recent indwelling Foley, if feasible, should be converted to a short period of CIC to allow for bladder cycling. Often, in these patients without a high suspicion of true poor compliance, normal compliance will be noted after a short period of CIC and/or bladder cycling. When documenting the interpretation of the UDS tracing, compliance is usually reported as normal or abnormal or can be listed as a calculated value as noted previously.

2.2.1.3 Contractions (Detrusor Overactivity)

Detrusor overactivity (DO) is defined as a urodynamic observation characterized by involuntary detrusor contractions during the filling phase which may be spontaneous or provoked. If there is a relevant neurologic lesion, it is deemed neurogenic DO. If there is no relevant neurologic lesion, it is deemed idiopathic DO [1]. It is important to ensure than any suspected detrusor overactivity is in fact accurate and not artifact. True detrusor overactivity is noted as a wavelike form on the P_{det} tracing along with a similar wavelike form on P_{ves} in the absence of "permission to void." Additionally, the interpreter must ensure that there is no dropout from the rectal/abdominal catheter (P_{abd}) that may artificially simulate a rise in detrusor pressure.

Often, patients will report an unintended or sudden urge to urinate which may or may not correlate with an IDC. It is key for the interpreter of the UDS tracing to be involved in the study as this helps identify artifact from true detrusor overactivity and can confirm if the DO replicates the patients presenting symptoms. Additionally, DO can be "stress induced" by strain or cough, so it is important to be aware of potential precipitating events both during the study and at home.

When documenting the interpretation of the UDS tracing, detrusor contractions during the filling phase are usually reported as absent ("stable filling"), present and suppressible, present with resulting detrusor overactivity incontinence, or terminal DO (DO-related incontinence resulting in emptying of the bladder) (Fig. 2.3). DO, which occurs at cystometric capacity and results in bladder emptying, is referred to as "terminal detrusor overactivity." An after contraction is a large amplitude rise in P_{det} occurring after the cessation of voiding. The clinical significance of this finding is unclear as it may represent catheter artifact or a true abnormality. While there is no defined high/low limit of rise in P_{det} to be considered DO, the definitive interpretation of low-amplitude DO (less than 5 cm H$_2$O) requires a high-quality UDS study [1].

2.2.1.4 Cystometric Capacity

Cystometric capacity is the volume in which "patients with *normal* sensation can no longer delay micturition" [1]. Cystometric capacity should not be confused with functional bladder capacity which is obtained from a voiding diary in conjunction with a post void residual. Cystometric capacity is typically less than the functional bladder capacity. There is no universally defined normal cystometric capacity, but typical values range from 370 to 540 mL ± 100 cm^3 [13]

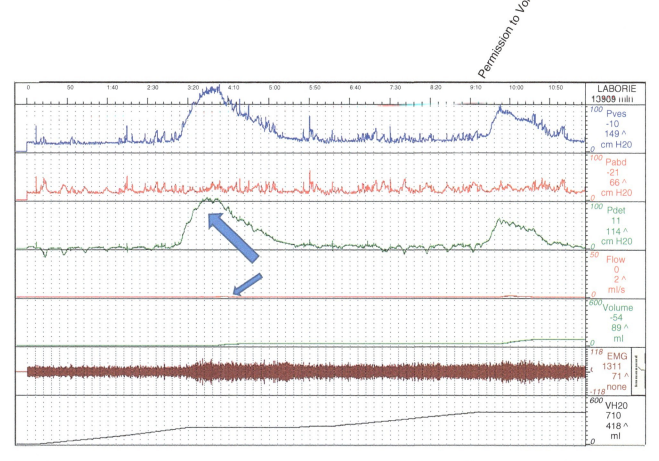

Fig. 2.3 Detrusor overactivity. The *arrows mark* detrusor overactivity with resulting leak. Note that detrusor overactivity and a normal detrusor contraction during voiding can look very similar. The key differentiation is the annotation of "permission to void"

(Fig. 2.4). Of note, the provider performing the UDS should ensure the patient is not experiencing an involuntary detrusor contraction which is generating the sensation such that they cannot delay micturition.

The filling rate of the bladder can also affect the cystometric capacity. Generally, a filling rate of 50–70 mL/min is used in adults [14]. This filling range allows for the test to be completed in a reasonable amount of time yet minimizes the artifacts related to overly rapid bladder filling [15]. A voiding diary suggestive of large/small bladder capacity can assist in determining if a faster/slower fill rate is more appropriate. When documenting the interpretation of the UDS tracing, cystometric capacity is usually reported in cm^3 or mL.

2.2.1.5 Continence

Continence refers to the presence or absence of urinary leakage during the UDS. The abdominal leak point pressure (ALPP), also known as cough leak point pressure or Valsalva leak point pressure, is defined as the lowest intravesical pressure at which urine leakage occurs because of increased abdominal pressure in the absence of a detrusor contraction [1].

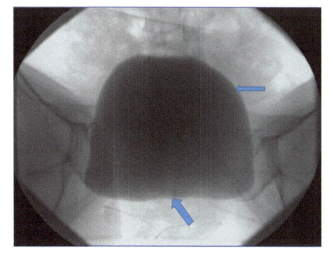

Fig. 2.4 Normal bladder at maximum cystometric capacity. The *narrow arrow marks* a smooth-walled bladder. The *thick arrow* demonstrates a closed bladder neck

While there is no universally accepted method to test ALPP, it is important to ensure that the leakage of urine reproduces the patient's symptoms.

If unable to reproduce a patient's symptomatic stress incontinence, provocative maneuvers (i.e., moving from sitting to standing) can be attempted. UDS can help differentiate stress-induced detrusor overactivity (Fig. 2.5) from true stress incontinence (Fig. 2.6). Having the patient cough or Valsalva may demonstrate stress-induced DO as their true etiology of incontinence. ALPP testing should not be performed during an involuntary detrusor contraction.

It is important to note that despite the small size of the urethral catheter, it can obstruct the bladder outlet masking urinary incontinence (i.e., bladder neck contracture). In patients with suspected stress urinary incontinence that is unable to be

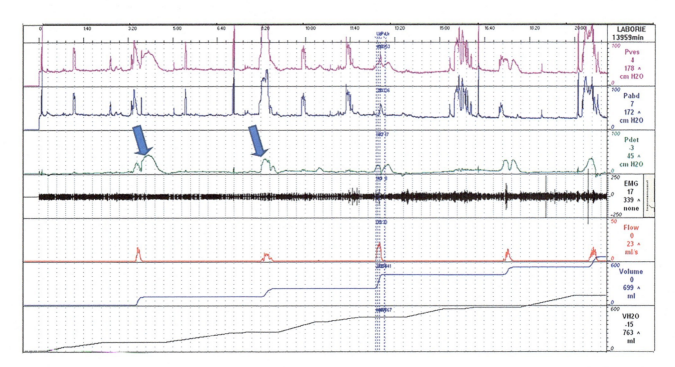

Fig. 2.5 Stress-induced detrusor overactivity. The *arrows* represent stress-induced detrusor overactivity with resultant urinary incontinence

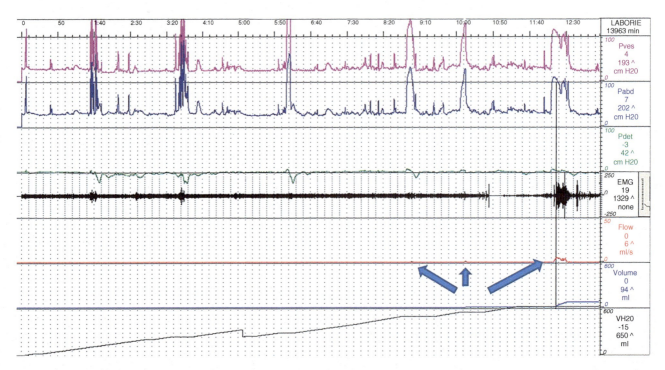

Fig. 2.6 Stress urinary incontinence. Note multiple cough and strain provocative maneuvers at low volumes with eventual stress urinary incontinence (*arrows*) at a volume of 570 mL at a pressure of 110 cm H_2O

reproduced during the UDS study, it has been suggested that the urethral catheter be removed and stress maneuvers repeated [16, 17]. Patients with advanced prolapse may have their prolapse reduced to rule out occult stress urinary incontinence which may be masked by urethral kinking from prolapse [18]. Lastly, it should be noted whether the urinary incontinence on the study reproduced the patients' presenting symptoms as the artificial circumstances of the UDS laboratory may result in spurious findings and thus erroneous interventions. When documenting the interpretation of the UDS tracing, incontinence is usually reported in absent (normal), present-stress incontinence, present-detrusor overactivity.

2.2.2 Emptying

The emptying phase begins when the bladder is filled to cystometric capacity, and in the absence of detrusor overactivity, the patient is given permission to void. Ideally, all questions regarding the patients filling phase should be addressed prior to initiating the emptying phase of the study.

2.2.2.1 Contractility

Once "permission to void" is given, the patient should initiate a volitional void. Urine flow should occur once the pressure generated by the detrusor overcomes the total bladder outlet resistance as the urethra closure forces diminish. There are no defined normative values for P_{det} during volitional voiding. In normal, unobstructed women, a detrusor contraction of 10–30 is generally considered normal. In normal, unobstructed men, a detrusor contraction of 30–50 is common [19, 20]. When considering "normal," it is important to assess both the magnitude and duration of the detrusor contraction in the context of the ability to empty the bladder (Fig. 2.7). It is important to note that some women will normally void via pelvic floor relaxation without generating a measurable detrusor contraction [21]. The lack of a detrusor contraction is not inherently abnormal as long as there is neither a neurologic etiology identified nor abnormal bladder emptying. While nomograms have been established to more objectively describe contractility in both men and women, these nomograms must be utilized in conjunction with clinical observations [22, 23].

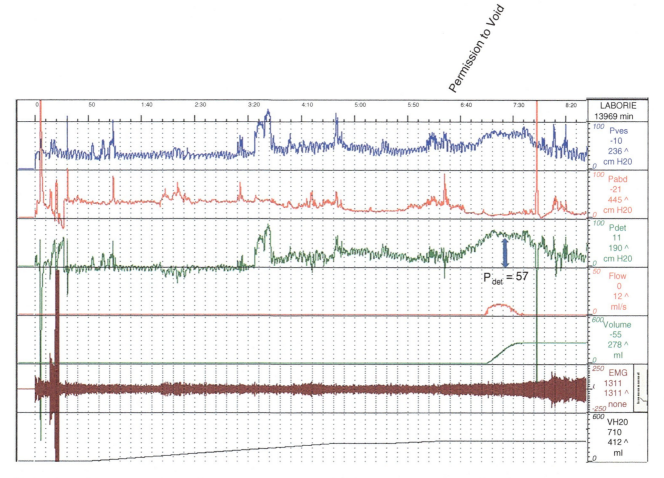

Fig. 2.7 Normal detrusor contractility. Note that compliance is normal. The apparent rise in P_{det} is artifactual and secondary to P_2 drop out. Similarly, note a small dropout in P_2 during voiding which makes the detrusor contraction appears to be artificially high

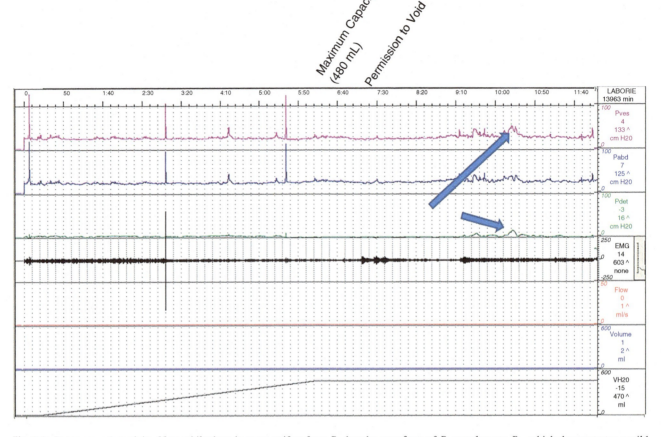

Fig. 2.8 Detrusor underactivity. Note while there is some artifact from P_2, but the waveform of P_1 correlates to P_{det} which demonstrates a mild poorly sustained detrusor contraction (*arrows*) that is unable to generate flow

Not infrequently, patients have a "shy bladder" or psychogenic inhibition and are unable to void during the emptying phase of the procedure. Allowing a faucet to run or giving the patient privacy in the UDS suite can often create a suitable environment for initiation of micturition. If the patient is still unable to void, performing the voiding phase on a noninvasive uroflow can still provide valuable information. When documenting the interpretation of the UDS tracing, contractility is usually reported as normal, absent, or underactive. There is no defined threshold for underactivity, but rather contractility is assessed in the context of the bladder's ability to empty appropriately and in most cases is related to the residual outlet resistance during the void (Fig. 2.8).

2.2.2.2 Coordination

The first recordable event in micturition is electrical silence of the pelvic floor EMG. Thus, coordination of voiding requires that the smooth and striated sphincters relax and open just prior to the onset of the detrusor contraction. During a normal void, the bladder neck and sphincter should remain open for the entire voiding period (Fig. 2.9). When increased EMG activity is seen or a lack of opening of the bladder outlet is noted on video urodynamics, a pathologic condition may exist.

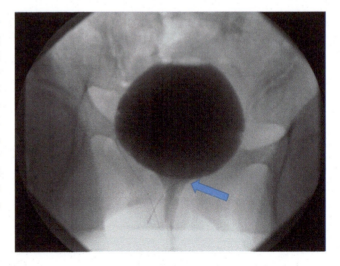

Fig. 2.9 Normal open bladder neck during voiding

If there is a lack of coordination in a patient without a known neurologic condition, consideration of a spinal condition may warrant referral to a neurologist. Lack of coordination in voiding may be seen in conditions such as detrusor external sphincter dyssynergia (DESD) and dysfunctional voiding (Fig. 2.10). However, apparent but artifactual unco-

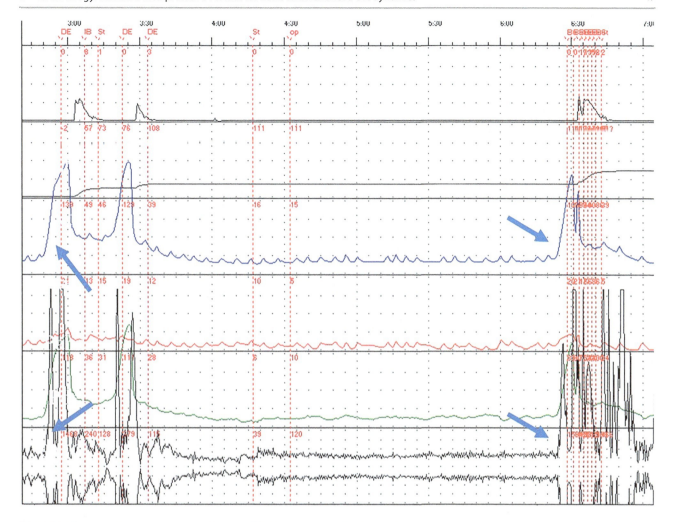

Fig. 2.10 Detrusor sphincter dyssynergia. Note the EMG flare begins at the time of the void

ordinated voiding may be seen in patients with pain related to the urethral catheterization for the UDS study. In such suspected cases, it is important to review the noninvasive (unintubated) uroflowmetry flow pattern to rule out catheter-related pain artifact resulting in an aberrant uroflow [24].

When documenting the interpretation of the UDS tracing, coordination is usually reported as coordinated or uncoordinated.

2.2.2.3 Complete Emptying

As noted previously, just prior to beginning the UDS study, the patient is catheterized for a PVR. At the conclusion of the study, a second PVR is calculated by subtracting the voided volume in the uroflow transducer from the infused volume. Emptying can be one of the more difficult parameters to accurately reproduce during urodynamics. Micturition is typically a private event which can be hard to replicate in a urodynamics lab. Urodynamics requires multiple transducers to be placed, two of which are invasive (vesical and rectal) and may result in pain and thus suppression of the micturition reflex. Additionally, the other individuals in the UDS laboratory—there is often a technician performing the study as well as a fluoroscopy technician in the room—may induce psychogenic inhibition due to voiding in front of others.

Complete emptying is defined by the lack of a significant post void residual (PVR). However, there is no universally accepted cutoff for a normal/abnormal PVR in either men or women. Typically, in men a PVR less than 50–100 mL is considered adequate bladder emptying, while a PVR greater than 200 mL is considered abnormal [25] (Fig. 2.11). In one study the median PVR was 19 mL and almost all women had a post void residual volume of less than 100 mL [26]. When documenting the interpretation of the UDS tracing, complete emptying is usually reported as normal or abnormal. Typically, the PVR is also reported in mL.

2.2.2.4 Clinical Obstruction

Clinical obstruction, also referred to as bladder outlet obstruction (BOO), is defined by the relationship between bladder pressure during voiding and urine flow. BOO is generally defined as high voiding pressure and low urine flow but may also occur in the setting of detrusor underactivity in

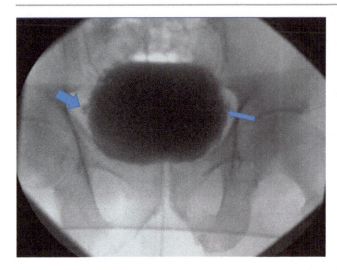

Fig. 2.11 Irregular bladder in a man with a large post void residual. The trabeculated bladder (*thin arrow*) with small right-sided diverticulum (*thick arrow*)

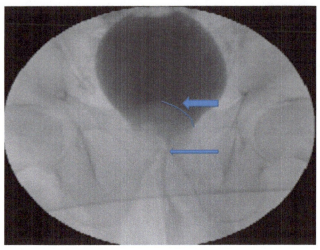

Fig. 2.12 Benign prostatic obstruction. Note the minimal contrast in obstructed prostatic urethra (*thin arrow*) and the "sunrise" sign filling defect from median lobe of the prostate (*thick arrow*)

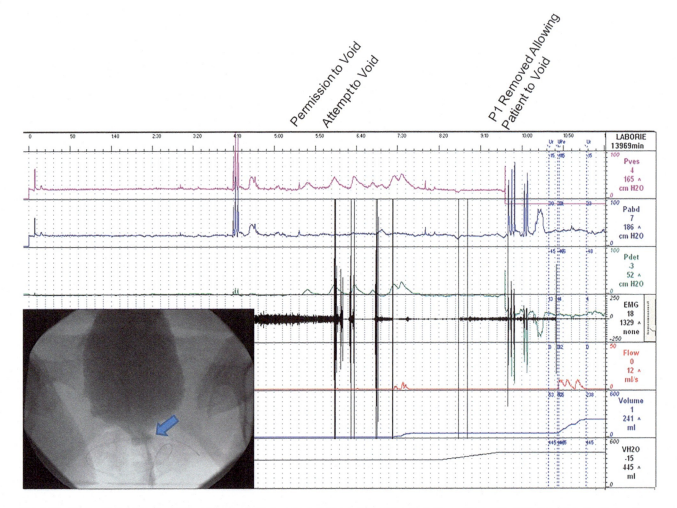

Fig. 2.13 Obstructing midurethral sling. Abrupt cutoff of contrast at obstructing midurethral sling with proximal dilation of urethra (*arrow*)

which the voiding pressure may be attenuated. BOO can result from a variety of causes. In men prostatic obstruction (Fig. 2.12), urethral stricture, and bladder neck contractures are common etiologies. In women, the most common cause is probably iatrogenic due to prior SUI surgery or vaginal prolapse (Fig. 2.13). Other less common causes include primary bladder neck obstruction (Fig. 2.14) and dysfunctional voiding. While there are multiple nomograms to assess

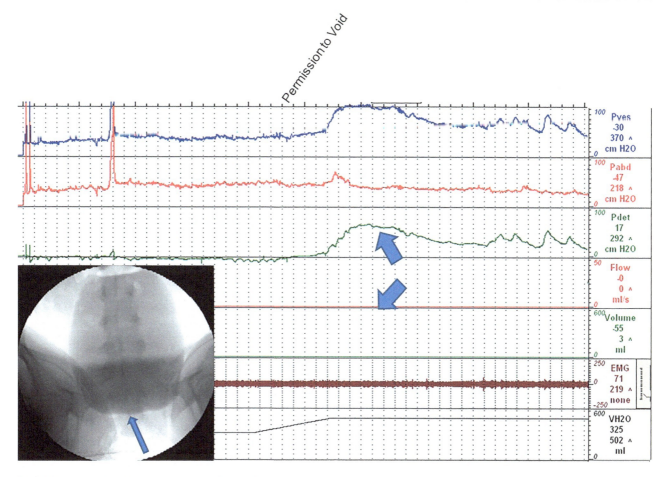

Fig. 2.14 Primary bladder neck obstruction. The *thick arrows* denote a strong detrusor contraction without flow. The *thin arrow* demonstrates a closed bladder neck during attempt to void

bladder outlet obstruction, there is no accepted definition of obstruction, nor dominate nomogram to establish the diagnosis [27, 28]. While nomograms have been established to more objectively describe obstruction, these nomograms must be utilized in conjunction with clinical observations [22, 23].

When documenting the interpretation of the UDS tracing, clinical obstruction is usually reported as unobstructed, equivocal, or obstructed.

2.3 Conclusion

Urodynamics plays an important role in evaluating lower urinary tract function. Over the course of the last few decades as urodynamicists gained an evolving understanding of the lower urinary tract, great efforts were undertaken to develop standardized testing formats and terminology to allow for reproducible results that can be communicated to other healthcare providers. As part of this, we feel that the use of the "9 Cs" provides a simple and concise means to evaluate and report upon the large amount of data generated by urodynamics testing.

References

1. Abrams P, Cardoza L, Fall M, Griffiths D, Rosier P, Ulmsten U, Kerrekroeck P, Victor A, Wein A. The standardization of terminology of lower urinary tract function: report from the standardization sub-committee of the international continence society. Neurourol Urodyn. 2002;21:167–78.
2. Perez LM, Webster GD. The history of urodynamics. Neurourol Urodyn. 1992;11(1):1–21.
3. Rovner ES, Koski ME. Rapid and practical interpretation of urodynamics. Philadelphia: Springer; 2014.
4. Lucia van Leijsen SA, Kluivers KB, Mol BW, et al. Value of urodynamics before stress urinary incontinence surgery: a randomized controlled trial. Obstet Gynecol. 2013;121(5): 999–1007.
5. Clement KD, Lapitan MCM, Omar MI, Glazener CMA. Urodynamic studies for the management of urinary incontinence in children and adults. Cochrane database of systematic reviews 2013; 10:Art. No.CD003195.
6. Nager CW, Brubaker L, Litman HJ, Zyczynski HM, Varner RE, Amundsen C, Sirls LT, Norton PA, Arisco AM, Chai TC, Zimmern P, Barber MD, Dandreo KJ, Menefee SA, Kenton K, Lowder J, Richter HE, Khandwala S, Nygaard I, Kraus SR, Johnson HW, Lemack GE, Mihova M, Albo ME, Mueller E, Sutkin G, Wilson TS, Hsu Y, Rozanski TA, Rickey LM, Rahn D, Tennstedt S, Kusek JW, Gormley EA; Urinary Incontinence

Treatment Network. A randomized trial of urodynamic testing before stress-incontinence surgery. N Engl J Med. 2012;366(21):1987–97.
7. Wein A. Classification of neurogenic voiding dysfunction. J Urol. 1981;125:605–9.
8. Peter FWM, Rosier PFWM, Kuo HC, De Gennaro M, Kakizaki H, Hashim H, Van Meel TD, Hobson PT. Urodyanmics. In: Abrams P, Cardozo L, Khoury S, Wein A, editors. Incontinence. 5th ed. Arnheim, The Netherlands: ICUD—European Association of Urology; 2013.
9. Haylen B, de Ridder D, Freeman RM, Swift SE, Berghmans B, Lee J, Monga A, Petri E, Rizk DE, Sand PK, Schaer GN. An International Urogynecological Association (IUGA)/International Continence Society (ICS) joint report on the terminology for female pelvic floor dysfunction. Int Urogynecol J. 2010;21:5–26.
10. Stöhrer M, Goepel M, Kondo A, Kramer G, Madersbacher H, Millard R, Rossier A, Wyndaele JJ. The standardization of terminology in neurogenic lower urinary tract dysfunction: with suggestions for diagnostic procedures. International Continence Society Standardization Committee. Neurourol Urodyn. 1999;18(2):139–58.
11. McGuire EJ, Cespedes RD, O'Connell HE. Leak-point pressures. Urol Clin North Am. 1996;23:253–62.
12. McGuire EJ, Woodside JR, Borden TA, Weiss RM. Prognostic value of urodynamic testing in myelodysplastic patients. J Urol. 1981;126(2):205–9.
13. Rosier PFWM, Kuo H-C, De Gennaro M. Urodynamic testing. In: Abrams P, Cardozo Khoury A, Wein A, editors. Incontinence. 5th ed. Arnheim, The Netherlands: ICUD—European Association of Urology; 2013.
14. Abrams P, Blaivas JG, Stanton SL, Andersen JT. The standardization of terminology of lower urinary tract function. Produced by the International Continence Society Committee on Standardization of Terminology. World J Urol. 1989;6:233–45.
15. Scarpero HM, Kaufman MR, Koski ME, et al. Urodynamics best practices. AUA Update Series. 2009;28:9.
16. Maniam P, Goldman HB. Removal of transurethral catheter during urodynamics may unmask stress urinary incontinence. J Urol. 2002;167(5):2080–2.
17. Smith AL, Ferlise VJ, Wein AJ, Ramchandani P, Rovner ES. Effect of A 7-F transurethral catheter on abdominal leak point pressure measurement in men with post-prostatectomy incontinence. Urology. 2011;77(5):1188–93.
18. Chaikin DC, Groutz A, Blaivas JG. Predicting the need for anti-incontinence surgery in continent women undergoing repair of severe urogenital prolapse. J Urol. 2000;163(2):531–4.
19. Osman NI, Chapple CR, Abrams P, Dmochowski R, Haab F, Nitti V, Koelbl H, van Kerrebroeck P, Wein AJ. Detrusor underactivity and the underactive bladder: a new clinical entity? A review of current terminology, definitions, epidemiology, etiology, and diagnosis. Eur Urol. 2014;65(2):389–98.
20. Cucchi A, Quaglini S, Rovereto B. Proposal for a urodynamic redefinition of detrusor underactivity. J Urol. 2009;181(1):225–9.
21. Tanagho EA, Miller ER. The initiation of voiding. Br J Urol. 1970;42:175–83.
22. Oelke M, Rademakers KL, van Koeveringe GA. Detrusor contraction power parameters (BCI and W max) rise with increasing bladder outlet obstruction grade in men with lower urinary tract symptoms: results from a urodynamic database analysis. World J Urol. 2014;32(5):1177–83.
23. Abrams P. Bladder outlet obstruction index, bladder contractility index and bladder voiding efficiency: three simple indices to define bladder voiding function. BJU Int. 1999;84(1):14–5.
24. Nitti VW. Urodynamic and video-urodynamic evaluation of the lower urinary tract. In: Wein A, Kavoussi LR, Novick AC, et al., editors. Campbell-Walsh urology. 10th ed. Philadelphia: Elsevier Saunders; 2012. p. 1847–70.
25. Agency for Health Care Policy and Research. Clinical practice guideline: urinary incontinence in adults. AHPCR Pub. No. 96-0682. Rockville, MD: Dept of Health and Human Services (US), Agency for Health Care Policy and Research; 1996.
26. Gehrich A, Stany MP, Fischer JR, Buller J, Zahn CM. Establishing a mean postvoid residual volume in asymptomatic perimenopausal and postmenopausal women. Obstet Gynecol. 2007;110(4):827–32.
27. Griffiths CJ, Harding C, Blake C, McIntosh S, Drinnan MJ, Robson WA, et al. A nomogram to classify men with lower urinary tract symptoms using urine flow and noninvasive measurement of bladder pressure. J Urol. 2005;174(4 Pt 1):1323–6.
28. De Nunzio C, Autorino R, Bachmann A, Briganti A, Carter S, Chun F, Novara G, Sosnowski R, Thiruchelvam N, Tubaro A, Ahyai S. The diagnosis of benign prostatic obstruction: development of a clinical nomogram. Neurourol Urodyn. 2016;35(2):235–40.

Overactive Bladder: Non-neurogenic

Marisa M. Clifton and Howard B. Goldman

3.1 Introduction

Overactive bladder is a clinical diagnosis defined by the International Continence Society (ICS) as the presence of urinary urgency, usually accompanied by frequency and nocturia, with or without urgency urinary incontinence, in the absence of a urinary tract infection (UTI) or other obvious pathology. Urgency is the complaint of a sudden, compelling desire to urinate which is difficult to defer [1]. Urinary frequency is the number of voids per time period, and traditionally up to 7 voids per day (waking hours) was considered normal. However, this is highly variable [2]. Increased urinary frequency is the complaint that micturition occurs more frequently during waking hours than previously deemed normal by the patient. Thus, it is all relative to the prior perception of "normal" frequency of the patient. Urgency urinary incontinence is the involuntary leakage of urine associated with a sudden compelling desire to void. Ultimately OAB is a clinical diagnosis characterized by the presence of *bothersome* symptoms [1]. In patients with mixed urinary incontinence (both stress and urgency incontinence), it can sometimes be difficult to distinguish incontinence subtypes [3].

The evaluation of a patient with OAB should focus on symptom presentation and degree of bother associated with those symptoms. A patient with OAB may describe increased urinary frequency, urgency, nocturia, and possibly incontinence. It is important to distinguish urgency incontinence, or leakage associated with or proceeded by a strong urgency to void, from stress urinary incontinence—leakage that occurs with a rise in abdominal pressure such as with coughing, laughing, sneezing, jumping, or change in position. Many patients may have both forms of incontinence—mixed urinary incontinence. It is also imperative to assess bladder emptying by history and physical examination in order to exclude overflow urinary incontinence. If there is a suspicion of incomplete emptying, a noninvasive bladder scan should be performed to measure the post-void residual (PVR). Additionally, the use of validated questionnaires may be helpful in diagnosing incontinence. A detailed history is likely the most important piece of the diagnostic process necessary to diagnose OAB.

A detailed physical exam should be performed focusing on the lower abdomen and genitourinary system with some attention to assessing intact neurologic function. The bladder should not be palpable or painful on suprapubic exam, and the patient should have normal sensation in the lower abdomen, vaginal, and rectal regions. In women, a pelvic exam should be performed in the low lithotomy position with the use of a half speculum to assess not only the anterior but also the apical and posterior compartments to ensure no significant pelvic organ prolapse is present. The use of the Pelvic Organ Prolapse Quantification (POP-Q) system may be used to further characterize the patient's prolapse. The exam should note the presence of vaginal atrophy and voluntary pelvic floor muscle strength. A cough stress test may be performed to identify stress urinary incontinence. This test is performed with the patient initially in the supine position with a full bladder. The patient is asked to cough and the physician is able to note if there is any loss of urine. If the patient has a history of stress incontinence that is not observed, the patient should repeat the test in the standing position with at least 300 cm^3 in the bladder [4]. In men, it is important to perform a digital rectal examination to ensure there are no abnormalities of the prostate or anal sphincter.

Testing for patients who complain of OAB symptoms includes a urinalysis to ensure no infection or hematuria exists. In patients with positive leukocyte esterase and/or nitrates found on urine dipstick, the urine should be sent for culture and the patient should be treated accordingly. Patients with straightforward OAB may not need further evaluation; however, those with an elevated PVR or other concerning symptom may need UDS evaluation.

M.M. Clifton, M.D. • H.B. Goldman, M.D. (✉)
Department of Urology, Cleveland Clinic Foundation,
9500 Avenue/Q10-1, Cleveland, OH 44195, USA
e-mail: marisameyerclifton@gmail.com; goldmah@ccf.org

The typical urodynamic finding in a patient with idiopathic OAB is either bladder hypersensitivity or detrusor overactivity. In bladder hypersensitivity, the sensation of filling and the need to void occur at a much lower volume than in typical patients. Thus, the urge to void occurs much earlier during bladder filling than is normal. This urge to void occurs without any change in detrusor pressure—no detrusor overactivity. On the other hand, other patients may have bladder contractions represented by elevations in detrusor pressure during the filling phase—so called detrusor overactivity. Regardless, the symptom that the patient reports is urgency.

Urodynamic testing is not necessary in all patients with OAB but may be indicated in patients with the following risk factors, especially if surgical intervention is being considered: advanced age, history of previous continence surgery, symptoms suggestive of outlet obstruction or voiding dysfunction, elevated post-void residual, radiation to the pelvis, whenever the diagnosis of OAB is in question, as well as when the patient has a neurologic disease that can affect lower urinary tract function or contribute to abnormal sacral neurologic examination. Urodynamics are important in specific patient populations as these studies identify abnormalities other than overactive bladder. They can reveal occult stress urinary incontinence in patients with negative clinical stress tests, elucidate the source of insensate incontinence, determine obstruction during the voiding phase, identify changes in bladder compliance, as well as identify other pathophysiologic processes.

3.2 Case Studies

3.2.1 Patient 1: Detrusor Overactivity

3.2.1.1 History

The patient is a 64-year-old woman with no significant past medical history who presents with a long-standing history of urinary urgency incontinence. When she drinks coffee or alcohol, she will have to urinate every 5 min. She finds it difficult to travel. From a leakage standpoint, she has multiple episodes of UUI per day. She uses 5–6 pads per day. She urinates large amounts and empties to completion. Additionally, she complains of nocturia 4 or 5 times per night. She has previously tried behavioral modification, pelvic floor physical therapy, and multiple overactive bladder medications.

3.2.1.2 Physical Examination

General appearance: no acute distress
Psychologic: no signs of depression
Neurologic: normal gait and sensory examination
Cardiovascular: no labored breathing or extremity edema
Abdomen: soft, nontender, nondistended
Genitalia: mild vaginal atrophy and no SUI on examination.
No significant prolapse noted

3.2.1.3 Labwork/Other Studies

Urinalysis—negative
US PVR—15 mL

3.2.1.4 UDS

See Fig. 3.1.

Findings

Filling Phase
- First desire at 82 cm^3.
- Strong desire soon after.
- Multiple detrusor contractions at 160, 175, 189, 197, and 200 cm^3.
- Large amplitude detrusor contractions starting at a volume of 160 cm^3 with a maximum filling detrusor contraction pressure of 100 cm of H_2O
- Normal compliance throughout filling.
- No evidence of stress urinary incontinence despite coughs at 150 and 200 cm^3.
- EMG demonstrates activity during large DO event.

Voiding Phase
- Patient voids to completion with 200 cm^3 instilled and 210 cm^3 voided.
- Patient voids with an excellent flow with a maximum flow of 27.5 mL/s.

This urodynamic study shows a patient with early first desire at 82 cm^3 with a strong desire soon after. She has urodynamic detrusor overactivity while filling. Her compliance is normal throughout filling. She has a large detrusor contraction at a bladder volume of 200 cm^3. After this contraction dissipates, the patient is given permission to void. She empties to completion with a good flow and no evidence of obstruction.

3.2.1.5 Treatment Options

- Observation—as the patient is significantly bothered by her symptoms, this is not the optimal option.
- Trial of a different overactive bladder medication.
- Percutaneous tibial nerve stimulation (PTNS).
- Onabotulinum toxin A injections (100 units).
- Sacral neuromodulation.

3 Overactive Bladder: Non-neurogenic

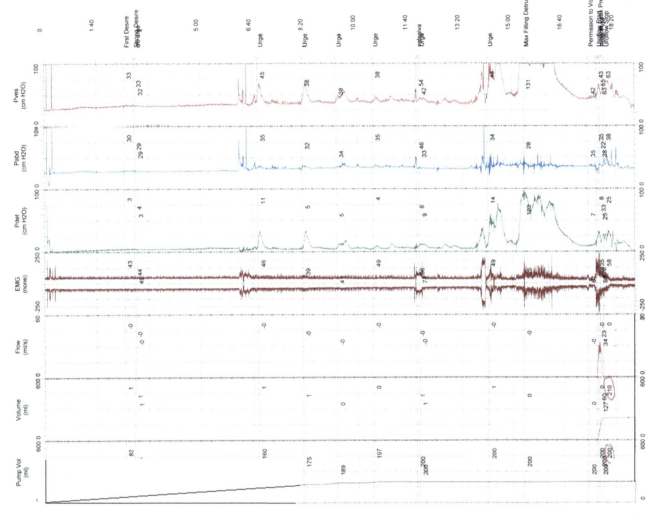

Fig. 3.1 Detrusor overactivity

3.2.2 Patient 2: Bladder Hypersensitivity

3.2.2.1 History

The patient is a 35-year-old woman with a history of obesity and GERD who complains of a 1-year history of worsening urinary frequency. She urinates every 30 min in the morning and then every hour during the afternoon. She complains of leakage but does not feel when it occurs and cannot tell if it happens with stress maneuvers. She notices intermittently that her underwear is damp and is unsure if this dampness is from urine. She has tried fluid management and some behavioral modification.

3.2.2.2 Physical Examination

General appearance: no acute distress, BMI 36
Psychologic: no signs of depression
Neurologic: normal gait and sensory examination
Cardiovascular: no labored breathing or extremity edema
Abdomen: soft, nontender, nondistended
Genitalia: no SUI on examination. No prolapse noted

3.2.2.3 Labwork/Other Studies

Urinalysis—negative
US PVR—0 mL

3.2.2.4 UDS

See Fig. 3.2.

Findings
  Filling Phase
- First desire at 44 cm^3
- Strong desire at 71 cm^3
- No DO

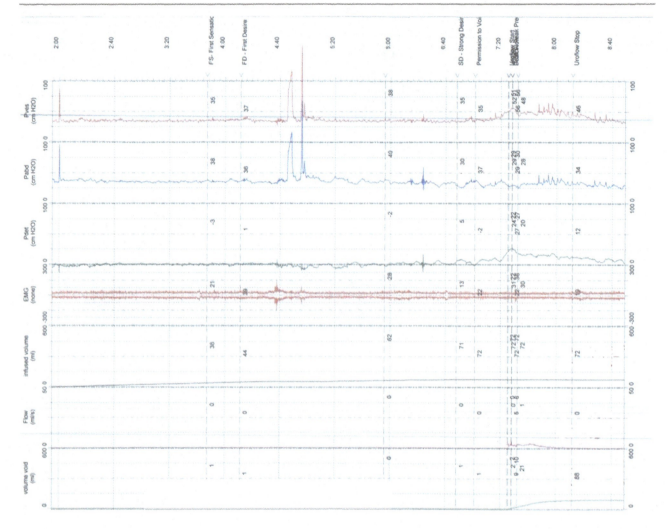

Fig. 3.2 Bladder hypersensitivity

- No SUI
- Normal compliance
- EMG normal

Voiding phase
- Patient voids to completion with 72 cm³ instilled and 88 cm³ voided
- Patient voids with a $P_{det}Q_{max}$ of 26.7 cm H$_2$O and a Q_{max} of 6.2 mL/s

The patient has an early first sensation and early first desire during filling. She also has an early strong desire at 71 cm³, indicating bladder hypersensitivity. However, she does not have urodynamic detrusor overactivity. Her compliance is normal during filling. When she voids, her pressure is high and her flow is low; however, the patient states her flow is usually much better than this. It is important to ask patients if their findings on UDS are typical of their symptoms. In this case, the patient usually voids with a much better force of stream.

3.2.2.5 Treatment Options
- Observation
- Behavioral modification
- Pelvic floor physical therapy
- Overactive bladder medications

If these are unsuccessful:

- PTNS
- Onabotulinum toxin A injections (100 units)
- Sacral neuromodulation

3.2.3 Patient 3: Bladder Outlet Obstruction with Detrusor Overactivity

3.2.3.1 History
The patient is a 53-year-old woman who underwent synthetic midurethral sling placement at an outside hospital for symptomatic stress predominant mixed urinary inconti-

nence. Subsequently, she developed worsening urgency and urgency incontinence requiring multiple pads per day. She denies leakage with cough, sneeze, or laugh. However, she leaks frequently with significant urge. She uses 2–3 pads per day. She reports urinary hesitancy and markedly diminished urinary stream since the time of surgery. She has nocturia twice per night. She has had no treatment for her incontinence after her midurethral sling placement.

3.2.3.2 Physical Examination

General appearance: no acute distress.
Psychologic: no signs of depression.
Neurologic: normal gait and sensory examination.
Cardiovascular: no labored breathing or extremity edema.
Abdomen: soft, nontender, nondistended.
Genitalia: no evidence of mesh erosion and negative stress test. Patient has stage I apical and anterior prolapse that is not bothersome to her.

3.2.3.3 Labwork/Other Studies

Urinalysis—negative
US PVR—90 mL
Cystoscopy—no evidence of mesh erosion, mild trabeculations throughout the bladder

3.2.3.4 UDS

See Fig. 3.3.

Findings

Filling Phase
- First desire at 71 cm^3
- Strong desire at 223 cm^3
- Detrusor contraction at 273 cm^3
- Normal compliance throughout filling
- No evidence of stress urinary incontinence

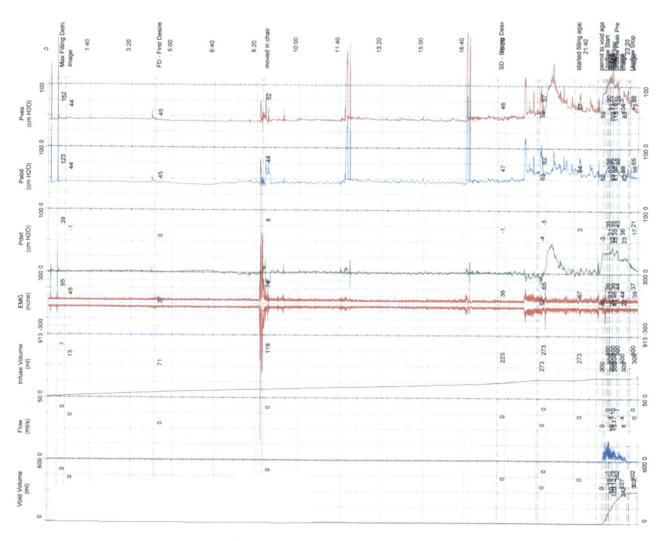

Fig. 3.3 Bladder outlet obstruction with detrusor overactivity

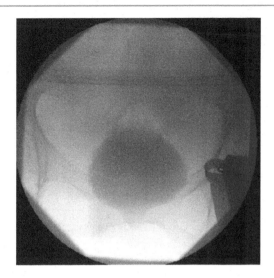

Fig. 3.4 Open bladder neck with mid-urethral narrowing on voiding phase of video urodynamics

Voiding Phase
- Elevated voiding pressures with a $P_{det}Q_{max}$ of 34 cm H_2O and a Q_{max} of 16 mL/s

The patient has an early first desire of 71 cm^3. Her strong desire occurs at 223 cm^3 and shortly thereafter during filling she has a detrusor contraction at 273 cm^3. She has normal compliance throughout filling without evidence of stress urinary incontinence. The patient is then given permission to void and has a voiding pressure of 34 at her maximum flow of 16 mL/s.

Because of concern regarding iatrogenic obstruction, video urodynamics was performed. The patient's bladder was noted to have a smooth contour while filling. However, when the patient was asked to void, her bladder neck was noted to be widely patent with a narrowing at the midurethra (Fig. 3.4). This is consistent with bladder outlet obstruction secondary to her synthetic midurethral sling.

3.2.3.5 Treatment Options
Sling incision: Iatrogenic obstruction from her sling is likely a significant contributor to her worsening OAB symptoms. Sling release will likely improve her urinary stream; however, all overactive bladder symptoms may not resolve. If bothersome OAB symptoms persist after sling release surgery, the patient may consider the following:

- Behavioral modification
- Pelvic floor physical therapy
- Overactive bladder medications
- PTNS
- Onabotulinum A toxin injections
- Sacral neuromodulation

3.3 Summary

Herein, we discussed the diagnosis of overactive bladder and reviewed the use of urodynamics in this patient population. Although the use of urodynamic studies for straightforward OAB is not recommended, they can be useful in patients with refractory OAB symptoms, symptoms suggestive of outlet obstruction or voiding dysfunction, elevated post-void residual, history of previous continence surgery, as well as in patients who have difficulty describing the type of incontinence they have.

References

1. Haylen BT, de Ridder D, Freeman RM, Swift SE, Berghmans B, Lee J, Monga A, Petri E, Rizk DE, Sand PK, Schaer GN. An International Urogynecological Association (IUGA)/International Continence Society (ICS) joint report on the terminology for female pelvic floor dysfunction. Neurourol Urodyn. 2010;29(1):4–20.
2. Fitzgerald MP, Brubaker L. Variability of 24-hour voiding diary variables among asymptomatic women. J Urol. 2003;169(1):207–9.
3. Gormley EA, Lightner DJ, Burgio KL, Chai TC, Clemens JQ, Culkin DJ, Das AK, Foster Jr HE, Scarpero HM, Tessier CD, Vasavada SP. Diagnosis and treatment of overactive bladder (non-neurogenic) in adults: AUA/SUFU guideline. J Urol. 2012;188(6):2455–63.
4. Nager CW. The urethra is a reliable witness: simplifying the diagnosis of stress urinary incontinence. Int Urogynecol J. 2012;23(12):1649–51.

Overactive Bladder: Neurogenic

Alana M. Murphy and Patrick J. Shenot

Abbreviations

AD	Autonomic dysreflexia
AUA	American Urological Association
CIC	Clean intermittent catheterization
CMG	Cystometrogram
DESD	Detrusor external sphincter dyssynergia
EMG	Electromyography
FDA	Federal Drug Administration
LUTS	Lower urinary tract symptoms
MS	Multiple sclerosis
OAB	Overactive bladder
PFS	Pressure flow studies
PMC	Pontine micturition center
PTNS	Percutaneous tibial nerve stimulation
PVR	Post-void residual
SCI	Spinal cord injury
SNM	Sacral neuromodulation
SUFU	Society of Urodynamics, Female Pelvic Medicine, and Urogenital Reconstruction
UUI	Urgency urinary incontinence

4.1 Introduction

Overactive bladder (OAB) refers to the bladder's inability to store urine. The hallmark of OAB is urgency, the sudden desire to pass urine which is difficult to defer. According to the International Continence Society, OAB syndrome is characterized by urgency, usually accompanied by urinary frequency and nocturia [1]. Patients with OAB may or may not have associated urgency urinary incontinence (UUI), defined as involuntary leakage of urine accompanied by a sense of urgency.

The clinical etiology of OAB is either idiopathic or secondary to a neurologic process. The term neurogenic OAB should be reserved for patients with a neurologic injury or disease state that leads to pathologic bladder innervation and subsequent OAB symptoms. Neurologic lesions above the pontine micturition center (PMC) that cause neurogenic OAB include cerebrovascular accidents, multiple sclerosis (MS), Parkinson's disease, and brain tumors. These lesions lead to a loss of detrusor inhibition and subsequent development of neurogenic OAB. Several lesions between the PMC and the termination of the spinal cord can cause neurogenic OAB, including MS, spinal cord injury (SCI), transverse myelitis, disk disease, and spinal stenosis. Patients with diabetes and OAB are also considered to have neurogenic OAB secondary to the nerve damage sustained as a result of glucose intolerance [2].

An initial assessment of patients with neurogenic OAB should include a comprehensive history and physical exam. Other urologic pathology can present alongside neurogenic OAB and may even cause similar symptoms. For this reason, patients should also be evaluated for diagnoses such as stress urinary incontinence, prostatic enlargement, or a urinary tract infection. A physical exam should include a focused neurologic assessment, including S2–S4 dermatomes, anal sphincter tone, and bulbocavernosus reflex. Since voiding dysfunction can also coexist in patients with neurogenic OAB, a post-void residual (PVR) volume should be performed, and a baseline upper tract radiologic evaluation can be obtained. Measurement of serum creatinine and calculation of glomerular filtration rate should be performed in patients with risk of upper tract impairment.

The American Urological Association (AUA) and Society of Urodynamics, Female Pelvic Medicine, and Urogenital Reconstruction (SUFU) published urodynamics guidelines in 2012 [3]. According to the guidelines, clini-

A.M. Murphy, M.D. (✉) • P.J. Shenot, M.D.
Department of Urology, Thomas Jefferson University Hospital, 1025 Walnut Street, Suite 1100, Philadelphia, PA 19107, USA
e-mail: alana.m.murphy.md@gmail.com; patrick.shenot@jefferson.edu

cians should perform a complex cystometrogram (CMG) during the initial evaluation of patients with relevant neurologic conditions with or without lower urinary tract symptoms (LUTS). Measurement of PVR, pressure flow studies (PFS), and electromyography (EMG) should also be performed in all patients with neurologic lower urinary tract dysfunction. These studies should also be performed as part of ongoing follow-up and can even be considered for patients with neurologic diagnoses that lack a direct correlation with LUTS. When available, the addition of fluoroscopy can provide important information regarding structural anomalies of the lower urinary tract and ureters.

In our practice, patients known or suspected to have neurogenic lower urinary tract dysfunction undergo a complete urodynamic evaluation (CMG, EMG, PFS, PVR, and fluoroscopy) at baseline. If applicable, the urodynamic evaluation is delayed until after resolution of spinal shock (approximately 12 weeks). The optimal frequency of urodynamics in neurogenic lower urinary tract dysfunction remains unknown. Our protocol is to conduct repeat evaluations to monitor patients at risk for upper tract deterioration. Our spinal cord injury patients are studied every other year if their urodynamic parameters have been stable in the past. Patients with impaired compliance and elevated bladder storage pressures undergo more frequent evaluations until we achieve the goal of low-pressure urine storage. Repeat urodynamics are also conducted in neurogenic patients to investigate treatment failures and when clinical complaints change.

When performing urodynamics on SCI patients, special consideration should be given to autonomic dysreflexia (AD). As a potentially life-threatening clinical emergency, AD is defined as an increase in systolic blood pressure by at least 20 mmHg from baseline [4]. AD is the most common in SCI patients with lesions at or above T6 and is often accompanied by bradycardia. AD can be "silent" or accompanied by symptoms, such as headache, anxiety, flushing, nausea, and sweating above the level of the SCI. Patients at risk to develop AD should undergo blood pressure monitoring during urodynamics, since bladder distension during CMG has been shown to trigger AD in 37–78 % of cases [5]. Our protocol is also to start with a slow bladder filling rate of 10 mL/min with patients at risk for AD. If vital signs remain stable over the first 5 min of the filling phase, we then gradually increase the filling rate. If AD develops, then the bladder should be emptied immediately, and shorter-acting antihypertensive medications, such as nifedipine and nitrates, should be administered with continued vital sign monitoring until vital signs stabilize. Although we always have immediate access to short-acting antihypertensive medications in our urodynamic suite, we do not routinely administer prophylactic antihypertensive medication for our neurogenic patients.

While neurogenic OAB can be diagnosed solely on clinical symptoms, urodynamics allows for the observation and diagnosis of specific facets of OAB. A urodynamic tracing can be segregated into a filling and a voiding phase. The urodynamic components of OAB are isolated to the filling phase, and emphasis should be placed on this portion of the test during the evaluation of neurogenic OAB. Patients with intact sensory innervation may demonstrate bladder oversensitivity, which is the early desire to void at a low bladder volume. Bladder oversensitivity, previously referred to as "sensory urgency," should be diagnosed when there is no associated abnormal increase in detrusor pressure [1]. Filling CMG may also demonstrate neurogenic detrusor overactivity, involuntary detrusor contractions that are either phasic or terminal [1]. Neurogenic detrusor overactivity may or may not be associated with a sensation of urgency or UUI. Similar to idiopathic cases of OAB, patients with neurogenic OAB may fail to complain of urgency or demonstrate detrusor overactivity during a urodynamic evaluation. Lack of bladder oversensitivity or detrusor overactivity should be viewed as a shortcoming of urodynamics to capture day-to-day bladder behavior and not a reason to revoke a clinical diagnosis of neurogenic OAB. Patients with neurogenic OAB may also demonstrate evidence of detrusor underactivity, a detrusor contraction of reduction strength and/or duration, during the voiding phase [1, 6].

There is evidence to suggest that neurogenic detrusor overactivity can be distinguished from idiopathic detrusor overactivity on a filling CMG [7, 8]. In a study by Lemack and colleagues, the urodynamic characteristics for 54 women with neurogenic detrusor overactivity secondary to MS were compared to 42 women with idiopathic detrusor overactivity. Compared to women with idiopathic detrusor overactivity, women with neurogenic detrusor overactivity had a greater amplitude for both their first overactive contraction (28.3 cm H_2O versus 20.5 cm H_2O, $p=0.003$) and their maximum detrusor contraction (46.4 cm H_2O versus 30.8 cm H_2O, $p=0.002$). Using their own dataset, the authors calculated an 88 % positive predictive value when a threshold of 30 cm H_2O for the amplitude of the first overactive contraction was used to distinguish between neurogenic and idiopathic detrusor overactivity.

Treatment algorithms for neurogenic OAB should be tailored to minimize OAB symptoms, improve continence, and achieve a lower pressure storage reservoir that protects the upper tracts. Appropriate treatment regimens should minimize patient risks, maximize social acceptability of bladder habits, and account for patient mental status, motivation, and physical capabilities. First-line therapy for neurogenic OAB consists of behavioral medication in the form of fluid management, dietary adjustment, timed voiding, and urge suppression techniques. These behavioral modifications are only appropriate in isolation for patients with low-pressure storage based on urodynamics and no risk of upper tract impairment. Antimuscarinic and β-3 agonist medications remain the second-line therapy for neurogenic OAB [9, 10]. Despite favorable success rates for the reduction in OAB symptoms, a significant portion of patients started on pharmacologic treatment will require third-line therapies for neurogenic OAB due to a lack of efficacy, loss of efficacy, or intolerance to side effects.

Current third-line therapies include direct detrusor neuromodulation in the form of botulinum toxin, sacral neuromodulation (SNM) using the InterStim® device (Medtronic, Minnetonka, MN, USA), and percutaneous tibial nerve stimulation (PTNS) using the Urgent PC® device (Uroplasty, Minneapolis, MN, USA). Since the Food and Drug Administration (FDA) approved the use of onabotulinumtoxinA for the treatment of neurogenic OAB in 2011, direct detrusor neuromodulation has gained considerable traction as the second-line treatment modality of choice for patients with neurogenic OAB. A recent review of prospective, randomized control trials demonstrates an improvement in continence rates (19–89 %), reduced storage pressures, and increased bladder capacities when onabotulinumtoxinA is utilized for neurogenic OAB [11]. The length of efficacy ranged from 6 to 9 months. Studies have also demonstrated the efficacy of SNM [12] and PTNS [13] for neurogenic OAB. PTNS is an office-based treatment easily used as a stand-alone treatment modality or an adjunct to OAB medication in the neurogenic population. While botulinumtoxin and PTNS have been readily applied to the management of neurogenic OAB, the practical application of SNM remains more controversial. Despite evidence supporting the safety of undergoing magnetic resonance imaging (MRI) with a 1.5 T magnet and an implanted InterStim® device [14, 15], Medtronic continues to limit their endorsement to only head imaging, and many radiology facilities will not perform MRI imaging caudad to the head if the patient has an InterStim® device [16]. In patients with neurogenic OAB who require periodic MRI imaging, this poses a challenge.

If third-line therapies fail, then a fourth-line therapy would involve augmentation cystoplasty in patients willing to perform self-catheterization. Although rates of augmentation cystoplasty have decreased in recent years, long-term studies indicate that patients undergoing augmentation cystoplasty continue to have reduced intravesical pressures, improved continence, and high rates of satisfaction [17].

4.2 Case Studies

4.2.1 Patient 1

4.2.1.1 History

The patient is a 39-year-old man with a past medical history significant for a T6 spinal cord injury secondary to a motor vehicle accident 7 years ago. He is a paraplegic who initially performed clean intermittent catheterization 4 times per day following his spinal cord injury. Approximately 2 years after his injury, he stopped performing self-catheterization due to his concern regarding recurrent urinary tract infections. For the past 5 years, he has managed his bladder with reflexive voiding into an adult diaper. Since he stopped self-catheterization, he has not experienced recurrent urinary tract infections. However, he now presents complaining of bothersome urgency urinary incontinence, which has required him to increase his adult diaper use from 3 to 6 diapers per day.

He denies any history of hematuria, flank pain, or known nephrolithiasis. He has had poor erections since the time of his spinal cord injury and is unable to participate in sexual activity. Finally, he has bowel movements every other day with the aid of stool softeners and laxatives.

4.2.1.2 Physical Examination

General: alert, oriented, and in no apparent distress. Wheelchair bound.
Abdomen: soft, nontender, and nondistended. No palpable bladder. No costovertebral tenderness bilaterally. No surgical scars.
Genitourinary: circumcised phallus with orthotopic meatus. Bilateral descended testes with no evidence of mass or edema. Digital rectal exam revealed a smooth 1+ prostate.
Neurologic: spastic paralysis of bilateral lower extremities. Intact bulbocavernosus reflex.
Bladder scan: 75 mL.

4.2.1.3 Labwork/Other Studies

Serum creatinine: 0.8 mg/dL
Renal and bladder ultrasound: symmetric kidneys with no hydronephrosis and no evidence of calculi or renal scarring, uniform thickening of bladder wall

4.2.1.4 UDS

See Fig. 4.1.

Findings

The urodynamic tracing demonstrates the filling phase. The patient's bladder was emptied by catheterization after he was unable to void; therefore, no PFS is included. The first evidence of neurogenic detrusor overactivity was noted at a bladder volume of 120 mL. The amplitude of detrusor contraction was >100 cm H_2O (Laborie urodynamic machines are usually not accurately calibrated above a contraction strength of 100 cm H_2O). The type of neurogenic detrusor overactivity was phasic. The increased EMG activity during each episode of detrusor overactivity was suggestive of detrusor external sphincter dyssynergia (DESD). Small volume UUI was demonstrated with each detrusor contraction (not registered on the flow curve but noted by the clinician performing the evaluation). The compliance was within normal limits at this low bladder capacity.

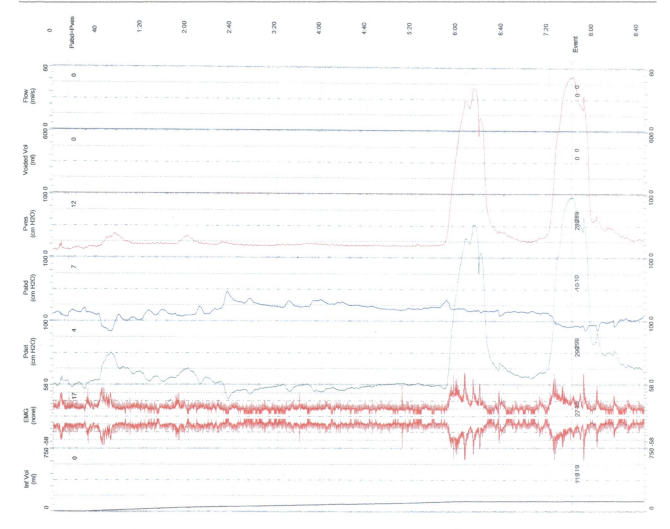

Fig. 4.1 Urodynamic tracing for 39-year-old man with T6 SCI

The corresponding fluoroscopy images demonstrated evidence of detrusor trabeculation with bilateral bladder diverticula (Fig. 4.2). There was no vesicoureteral reflux seen on this exam. Although no voiding phase was captured, the bladder trabeculation and bladder diverticula suggest high-pressure voiding consistent with DESD.

4.2.1.5 Treatment Options

In order to avoid high-pressure voiding and to improve his urinary incontinence, the patient was taught to perform clean intermittent catheterization and was placed on a daily antimuscarinic. Intradetrusor injection of onabotulinumtoxinA would be an appropriate treatment modality to add to CIC if he continues to have urinary incontinence between catheterizations. Augmentation cystoplasty would be reserved for refractory UUI after he had failed onabotulinumtoxinA treatment.

4.2.2 Patient 2

4.2.2.1 History

The patient is a 64-year-old woman with a past medical history significant for hypertension and hypothyroidism. Approximately 1 year ago, she began to experience a gait disturbance and a hand tremor. She developed a shuffling gait and increased limb rigidity. Her mobility was significantly impaired and her family had suggested she start to use a rolling walker. She also began to complain of urinary urgency, frequency, and worsening urinary incontinence. Although she had had infrequent episodes of stress urinary incontinence for many years, she began to wear pads on a daily basis due to urinary incontinence associated with urgency and not enough warning time to get to the bathroom. She does not complain of difficulty emptying her bladder. She admits that she does not

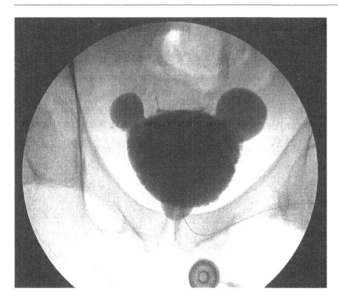

Fig. 4.2 Fluoroscopic image from filling phase for 39-year-old man with T6 SCI demonstrating bladder diverticula

keep herself well hydrated, but she has a habit of sipping on coffee throughout the day. Her neurologist has diagnosed her with Parkinson's disease and has started her on carbidopa/levodopa. She presents to her urologist since her worsening incontinence is having a negative impact on her quality of life.

4.2.2.2 Physical Examination

General: alert, oriented, and in no apparent distress. Ambulating with assistance of family member. Mild bilateral hand tremor

Abdomen: soft, nontender, and nondistended. No palpable bladder. No costovertebral tenderness bilaterally. Laparoscopic port site scars from previous cholecystectomy

Genitourinary: evidence of postmenopausal vaginal atrophy. Urethral hypermobility but no urinary incontinence with Valsalva maneuvers. No pelvic organ prolapse

Neurologic: cogwheel rigidity of bilateral lower extremities. Intact perineal sensation and bulbocavernosus reflex

Bladder scan: 30 mL after void

4.2.2.3 Labwork/Other Studies

Serum creatinine: 0.6 mg/dL

Renal and bladder ultrasound: symmetric kidneys with no hydronephrosis and no evidence of calculi or renal scarring, normal appearing bladder

4.2.2.4 UDS

See Fig. 4.3.

Findings

A slow infusion rate of 10 mL/min was used to minimize the provocative nature of bladder infusion. Her first bladder sensation was noted at only 13 mL. Starting at a low bladder volume of approximately 20 mL, the patient began to demonstrate phasic neurogenic detrusor overactivity. The maximum amplitude of detrusor contraction was 55 cm H_2O, and the patient experienced associated UUI with each episode of detrusor overactivity. The increased EMG activity during each episode of detrusor overactivity is consistent with a guarding reflex.

A cystoscopy performed after her urodynamic evaluation revealed an open bladder neck at rest and minimal bladder trabeculation (Fig. 4.4).

4.2.2.5 Treatment Options

In order to address her urinary urgency, frequency, and UUI, she was initially counseled regarding behavioral modification with limitation of her daily caffeine intake and improvement in her hydration status. She was also started on an anti-muscarinic medication. Due to her rapid impairment in gait and open bladder neck at rest, her urologic evaluation was reviewed with her neurologist and consideration was given to the diagnosis of multiple system atrophy.

4.3 Summary

Neurogenic overactive bladder (OAB) is characterized by urinary urgency usually accompanied by urinary frequency. Urgency urinary incontinence may or may not be present. The term neurogenic OAB should be reserved for patients with a neurologic injury or disease state that leads to OAB symptoms. The initial assessment of patients with neurogenic OAB should include a comprehensive history and physical exam, including a focused neurologic exam. In most cases, a urodynamic evaluation should be conducted to provide a baseline functional assessment and to identify potential threats such as high-pressure storage and subsequent upper tract risk. In order to provide a comprehensive assessment, urodynamics for patients with neurogenic OAB should include a cystometrogram, electromyography, pressure flow study, post-void residual urine measurement, and fluoroscopy when available. Special precautions should be taken for patients at risk for autonomic dysreflexia during bladder filling. Treatment modalities for neurogenic OAB include behavioral changes, OAB medications, various forms of neuromodulation, and augmentation cystoplasty in refractory cases.

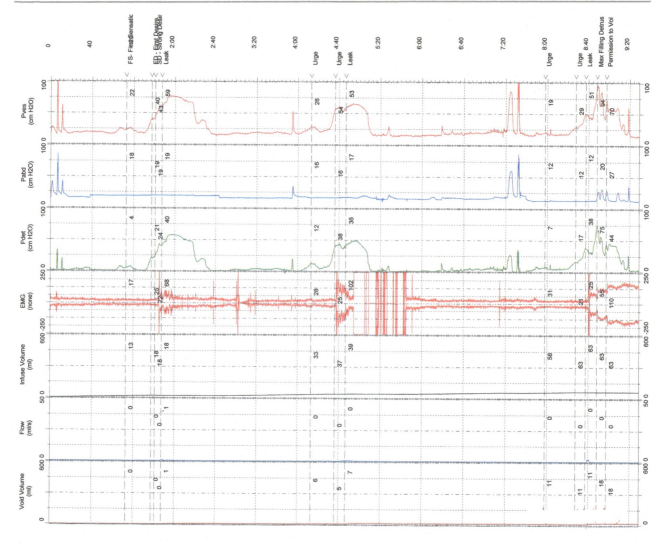

Fig. 4.3 Urodynamic tracing for 64-year-old woman with Parkinson's disease

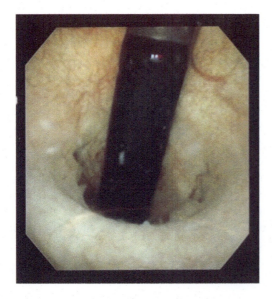

Fig. 4.4 Retroflexed cystoscopic image from 64-year-old woman with Parkinson's disease demonstrating open bladder neck

References

1. Haylen BT, de Ridder D, Freeman RM, Swift SE, Berghmans B, Lee J, et al. An International Urogynecological Association (IUGA)/International Continence Society (ICS) joint report on the terminology for female pelvic floor dysfunction. Neurourol Urodyn. 2010;29:4–20.
2. Golabek T, Kiely E, O'Reilly B. Detrusor overactivity in diabetic and non-diabetic patients: is there a difference? Int Braz J Urol. 2012;38:652–9.
3. American Urological Association/Society of Urodynamics Female Pelvic Medicine and Urogenital Reconstruction. Adult urodynamics: AUA/SUFU guideline. 2012. https://www.auanet.org/common/pdf/education/clinical-guidance/Adult-Urodynamics.pdf.
4. Krassioukov AV, Biering-Sorensen F, Donovan W, Kennelly M, Kirshblum S, Krogh K, et al. International standards to document remaining autonomic function after spinal cord injury. J Spinal Cord Med. 2012;35:201–10.
5. Liu N, Zhou M, Biering-Sorensen F, Krassioukov AV. Iatrogenic urological triggers of autonomic dysreflexia: a systematic review. Spinal Cord. 2015;53:500–9.
6. Natsume O. Detrusor contractility and overactive bladder in patients with cerebrovascular accidents. Int J Urol. 2008;15(6):505–10.

7. Gray R, Wagg A, Malone-Lee JG. Differences in detrusor contractile function in women with neuropathic and idiopathic detrusor instability. BJU Int. 1997;80:222–6.
8. Lemack GE, Frohman EM, Zimmern PE, Hawker K, Ramnarayan P. Urodynamic distinctions between idiopathic detrusor overactivity and detrusor overactivity secondary to multiple sclerosis. Urology. 2006;67(5):960–4.
9. Strohrer M, Blok B, Castro-Diaz D, Chartier-Kastier E, Del Popolo G, Kramer G, et al. EAU guidelines on neurogenic lower urinary tract dysfunction. Eur Urol. 2009;56(1):81–8.
10. Nitti V, Auerbach S, Martin N, Calhoun A, Lee M, Herschorn S. Results of a phase III randomized trial of mirabegron in patients with overactive bladder. J Urol. 2013;189(4):1388–95.
11. Linsenmeyer TA. Use of botulinum toxin in individuals with neurogenic detrusor overactivity: state of the art review. J Spinal Cord Med. 2013;36(5):402–19.
12. Peters KM, Kandagatla P, Killinger KA, Wolfert C, Boura JA. Clinical outcomes of sacral neuromodulation in patients with neurologic conditions. Urology. 2013;81(4):738–43.
13. Zecca C, Digesu GA, Robshaw P, Singh A, Elneil S, Gobbi C. Maintenance percutaneous posterior nerve stimulation for refractory lower urinary symptoms in patients with multiple sclerosis: an open label, multicenter, prospective study. J Urol. 2014;191(3):697–702.
14. Chermansky CJ, Krlin RM, Holley TD, Woo HH, Winters JC. Magnetic resonance imaging following InterStim®: an institutional experience with imaging safety and satisfaction. Neurourol Urodyn. 2011;30(8):1486–8.
15. Elkelini MS, Hassouna MM. Safety of MRI at 1.5 Tesla in patients with implanted sacral nerve stimulator. Eur Urol. 2006;50(2):311–6.
16. Medtronic. Medtronic InterStim® therapy: information for prescribers. Minneapolis: Medtronic, Inc.; 2014. http://manuals.medtronic.com/wcm/groups/mdtcom_sg/@emanuals/@era/@neuro/documents/documents/contrib_218753.pdf.
17. Gurung PM, Attar KH, Abdul-Rahman A, Morris T, Hamid R, Shah PJ. Long-term outcomes of augmentation ileocystoplasty in patients with spinal cord injury: a minimum of 10 years follow up. BJU Int. 2012;109(8):1236–42.

Female Stress Urinary Incontinence

Nitin Sharma, Farzeen Firoozi, and Elizabeth Kavaler

5.1 Introduction

Stress urinary incontinence (SUI) is the involuntary leakage of urine during increases in abdominal pressure (i.e., coughing, sneezing, straining, etc.) in the absence of a detrusor contraction [1]. Women typically develop SUI due to pelvic floor muscle weakening and a subsequent loss of urethral support. Pregnancy, vaginal childbirth, repetitive pelvic stress, as well as sphincteric atrophy from aging are often implicated as contributing factors for this condition which can affect up to 30 % of postpartum women [2]. The diagnosis of stress urinary incontinence in women is typically made following a focused history and physical exam. In cases of pure stress incontinence, patients will describe episodes of urinary leakage during coughing, sneezing, straining, etc. These episodes of urinary leakage are often reproducible on clinical exam when a rise in intra-abdominal pressure is elicited (i.e., Valsalva maneuver or cough) and urine is seen leaking from the urethral meatus. Patients demonstrating SUI in this manner generally do not need additional workup such as urodynamics and can be offered surgical treatment (i.e., urethral sling) with non-inferior outcomes [3].

However, not all cases of stress urinary incontinence present this simply. Over 10 % of women with stress urinary incontinence are found to have stress-induced detrusor overactivity (DO), in which detrusor instability and leakage occur following repetitive increases in abdominal pressure [4]. Additionally, a significant proportion of females that present with SUI will have *mixed urinary incontinence*, in which involuntary leakage occurs due to urinary urgency as well as during rises in intra-abdominal pressure [5]. As a result, eliciting a voiding history and performing a urinary stress (cough) test may not be sufficient in evaluating these more complicated cases of SUI, particularly when treatment is often surgical and an accurate diagnosis is necessary.

As described earlier in this book, the utility of urodynamic testing is not clearly defined for the workup of many lower urinary tract symptoms (LUTS), and universal indications for its use, particularly with SUI, are not absolute. Therefore, urodynamics should be used discriminately by the clinician only when a question regarding the patient's condition cannot be answered definitively based on history and physical exam. Cases of pure stress incontinence demonstrated clearly on clinical exam via a positive stress (cough) test do not require urodynamic evaluation. However, complicated cases of SUI, such as those listed in Table 5.1, represent distinct variations in presentation from the index patient with pure SUI and can account for over 50 % of patients presenting with urinary incontinence [6]. Urodynamics in these instances offer an objective assessment of both detrusor and urethral functions which can help the clinician better understand the etiology of incontinence while also identifying possible confounding variables that may exist within the clinical picture. In this chapter, we will focus on these more complicated cases of stress urinary incontinence in which urodynamic testing is warranted for accurate diagnosis and treatment selection.

5.2 Mechanisms of SUI and Urodynamic Considerations

To begin, normal female urinary continence is achieved when the urethra maintains a greater pressure than the bladder during states of rest and activity. During bladder filling

Table 5.1 Complicated SUI: indications for urodynamic evaluation

Mixed urinary incontinence
Failed stress incontinence surgery
Existing pelvic organ prolapse without stress urinary incontinence

and during increases in abdominal pressure, the anterior vaginal wall and surrounding connective tissues and muscles, which comprise the female pelvic floor, compress the urethra. Urethral closure pressures are therefore elevated relative to the bladder pressures that are generated, and continence is maintained. Additionally, the urethral sphincter itself has an intrinsic closure mechanism that increases during exertion and further prevents urinary leakage.

Stress urinary incontinence occurs when these normal mechanisms of continence are compromised. Repetitive pelvic stress experienced throughout pregnancy or pelvic stress experienced during the course of prolonged labor, constipation, or chronic respiratory conditions can lead to significant weakening and disruption of the pelvic floor nerves and musculature. *Urethral hypermobility* often results in this setting when the pelvic floor musculature is unable to provide sufficient support and compress the urethra. The bladder neck and proximal urethra normally maintain a high retropubic position, and increases in intra-abdominal pressures are transmitted equally to the bladder and urethra [7]. However, when pelvic floor muscle laxity occurs, the bladder neck and urethra cannot maintain their normal anatomic position, and the bladder neck and urethra rotate posteriorly and descend caudally which can lead to reduced urethral closing pressures and urinary incontinence (Fig. 5.1). *Intrinsic sphincteric deficiency* (ISD) is a second mechanism that leads to female stress urinary incontinence. ISD is a condition in which the bladder neck and/or proximal urethra remains partially open at rest. Urinary incontinence in this case develops despite normal pelvic floor musculature and despite minimal or no urethral descent during stress. ISD is often seen in patients due to atrophy of the sphincteric muscles from aging or in patients with persisting SUI following urethral sling surgery. All patients with SUI are believed to have some degree of ISD [5].

One of the problems clinicians often face when evaluating patients with SUI is identifying the primary etiology of incontinence. While it is clear that SUI can occur secondary to urethral hypermobility as well as ISD, the distinction of the two is not clinically relevant in most cases since treatment is generally the same. Patients with pure stress incontinence seen during an office stress test can be treated successfully with a urethral sling regardless of whether ISD or urethral hypermobility is the primary cause of their incontinence. However, patients with mixed urinary incontinence or patients with prior incontinence surgery and continued leakage should be evaluated more thoroughly. These patients may have urge-predominant symptoms due to detrusor overactivity or may have continued ISD despite prior sling placement with leakage. Urodynamics therefore can serve as a valuable diagnostic tool for these more complicated cases of SUI.

Urodynamics provides important information regarding the functionality of the bladder as well as the quality of the bladder outlet. The most important urodynamic studies for patients with SUI are leak point or urethral pressure profiles, opening detrusor pressures, as well as filling cystometry. These studies provide important information regarding the competence of the urethral sphincter and can shed light on the relative importance of contributory factors (i.e., detrusor instability, small bladder capacity, etc.) that may also exist along with SUI. These studies provide crucial information that can influence treatment options and help predict overall outcomes particularly in cases of urge-predominant mixed urinary incontinence, prior failed urethral slings, and pelvic organ prolapse.

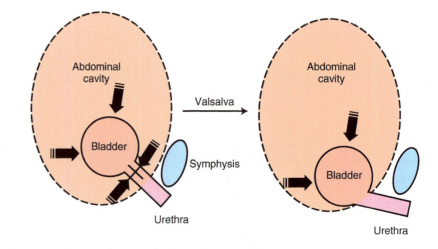

Fig. 5.1 Urethral hypermobility develops from loss of pelvic support surrounding the urethra. During increases in abdominal pressure, the bladder descends and urinary leakage can occur if urethral pressures are not maintained (Used with permission from Magon N, Kalra B, Malik S, Chauhan M. Stress urinary incontinence: what, when, why, and then what? J Midlife Health. 2011;2(2):57–64)

5.2.1 Leak Point Pressures

Leak point pressure, often referred to as *abdominal leak point pressure (ALPP)* or *Valsalva leak point pressure (VLPP)*, is the lowest abdominal pressure in which leakage is observed from the urethral meatus during cough or Valsalva in the absence of a detrusor contraction. Leak point pressure is the best measure of urethral sphincter strength, and it is used to evaluate the magnitude of abdominal force needed to drive urine across a closed urethral sphincter [8]. Patients with ALPP/VLPP less than 60 cm H_2O are considered to have urethral sphincteric incompetence or ISD. These patients when asked to cough or perform a Valsalva maneuver demonstrate urinary leakage from the urethral meatus at relatively low pressures.

For patients who are unable to reproduce SUI during urodynamics despite a clinical history of leakage, removing the urethral catheter can often unmask the patients' stress incontinence. Patient positioning is also an important factor when performing leak point pressure testing. Patients in a standing position may have lower leak point pressures than in a seated or lithotomy position. As a result, it is important that patient position be specified when performing the procedure and consistent during the entire examination. Urinary leakage determined by visual observation may also be challenging in some patients due to positioning, body habitus, or leakage of a low volume. Radiographic visualization of leakage may be useful in these cases but is less sensitive than direct visualization of the urethral meatus. Patients may also be asked to stand on an absorbent pad or to hold a towel at the labia to confirm urinary leakage.

5.2.2 Urethral Pressure Profile

Urethral pressure profile (UPP) is an alternative technique to evaluating the competence of the urethral sphincter. This test measures the urethral pressures along the full length of the urethra with the bladder at rest (Fig. 5.2). Specialized catheters with intravesical and intraurethral pressure transducers are required and pressures along the length of the urethra are recorded as the catheter is slowly withdrawn. The most important clinical measurement provided by a UPP is the *maximum urethral closure pressure (MUCP)* which is the difference between the maximum urethral and intravesical pressures. MUCP values less than 20 cm H_2O are considered to be diagnostic for ISD. Performing UPP is a more technically demanding test than calculating leak point pressures and consequently is less performed. Both UPP and leak point pressure testing evaluate the competence of the urethral sphincter.

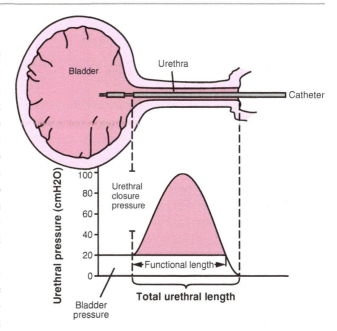

Fig. 5.2 Urethral pressure profile (UPP). Pressures along the length of the urethra allow the calculation of the length of the functional urethra relative to the total urethral length (Used with permission from Robinson D, Norton PA. Diagnosis and management of urinary incontinence. In: Mann W, Stovall TG editors. Gynecologic Surgery. New York: Churchill Livingstone; 1996. p. 704)

5.2.3 Cystometry

Filling cystometry is one of the most basic components of urodynamic testing for all forms of voiding dysfunction and can be a valuable tool when evaluating SUI, particularly in patients with mixed urinary incontinence. Bladder capacity, compliance, and detrusor activity are all important measures that provide information regarding the function of the bladder. Patients with uninhibited contractions during bladder filling or detrusor overactivity with SUI should be offered pharmacological treatment (i.e., anticholinergics) prior to considering surgical intervention. Detrusor contractions following provocative measures such as cough or Valsalva can also be identified during filling cystometry. Delayed urinary leakage may be seen in these cases resulting from *stress-induced detrusor overactivity* which is a different clinical entity than SUI. Additionally, patients with small capacity bladders or altered compliance can be identified during filling cystometry, and these patients can then be offered conservative management (i.e., biofeedback, pelvic floor exercise, medication) prior to surgical correction of their SUI. Filling cystometry is therefore one of the most important urodynamic tests in working up patients for SUI and should be carefully considered in all patients with complicated SUI prior to surgical planning.

5.3 Urodynamic Interpretations of Complicated SUI (Table 5.2)

5.3.1 Mixed Urinary Incontinence

Approximately 33 % of patients with urinary incontinence present with a mixed picture of both urge and stress incontinence [9]. If surgery is performed in these women without first addressing the urgency component, many of these patients will continue to be incontinent postoperatively. A thorough evaluation of a patient's incontinence is therefore important before any form of treatment is selected. Patients with predominantly urge incontinence should be managed first with behavioral modification, pelvic floor exercises, and/or medications. Urodynamics for these patients can be delayed in favor of these forms of conservative therapy only when urgency is the more bothersome symptom at the time of presentation. However, if urinary incontinence persists after initial conservative treatments have been offered, then urodynamics should be performed to further evaluate the patient's voiding dysfunction prior to any surgical intervention. Patients with stress-predominant mixed incontinence can forgo urodynamic evaluation all together if they are able to demonstrate stress incontinence on office evaluation. This was demonstrated in the VALUE trial in which women with stress-predominant urinary incontinence were randomized to either office evaluation or urodynamics prior to surgical treatment and were found to have equivalent outcomes [10].

For women with urge-predominant mixed incontinence, urodynamics offers important information about bladder function in both the filling and the emptying phases. The important findings on filling cystometry include bladder capacity, bladder compliance, coarse sensation, and detrusor overactivity. If the bladder capacity or compliance is reduced, there is evidence of detrusor overactivity, or if there are unstable contractions during filling, the urgency component will have to be addressed separately from the stress incontinence component. As mentioned, this can be done initially when patients present with predominantly urge incontinence or postoperatively for patients with mixed incontinence who continue to have urgency following sling placement. During the emptying phase of urodynamic studies, the degree of sphincteric or outlet resistance at the urethra can be evaluated by measuring leak point pressures or urethral pressure profiles. Patients with a poorly competent sphincter or ISD, as determined by a low ALPP or MUCP, will likely benefit from surgery to improve their incontinence, even in cases of detrusor overactivity. In these cases, patients may be offered surgical intervention for the treatment of SUI in addition to medical therapy for urinary urgency. An improvement in urgency symptoms has even been seen in some patients following midurethral sling placement alone [11, 12].

5.3.2 Failure of Prior Stress Incontinence Surgery

Synthetic midurethral slings have become the standard of care for the treatment of stress incontinence with success rates approaching 80 % in many studies [13]. However, as with any surgery, there is a subset of women who suffer from complications related to sling placement. Most of the postoperative complications following sling surgery involve voiding dysfunction with or without urinary obstruction [14]. In most cases, these complications can be resolved early in the postoperative period with temporary catheterization. However, in some cases urethral slings may be placed too tightly and lead to persistent obstructive urinary symptoms that necessitate a second surgery. In other cases, slings may improve sphincter competence but may indirectly exacerbate detrusor overactivity leading to worsening urgency with or without incontinence. Therefore, urodynamics can

Table 5.2 Urodynamic management for complicated cases of SUI

Problem being evaluated	Urodynamic values to focus on	How is treatment affected
Mixed incontinence (urge predominant)	Evaluate VLPP/MUCP	If DO is demonstrated, anticholinergics should be offered first
	Capacity	If SUI persists after conservative treatment for DO, then treat the SUI with MUS
	Compliance	If MUCP is very low despite DO, treat SUI first with MUS
	Coarse sensation	
	Detrusor overactivity (DO)	
Failed urethral sling	Evaluate for DO	If de novo DO is the problem, treat the DO with anticholinergics
	VLPP/MUCP	If urgency continues, revise the sling
	Opening detrusor pressure	If sling is found to be too tight, loosen then sling
	Pressure-flow	
Prolapse without SUI	Perform with pessary/prolapse reduction	Presence of occult SUI → urethral sling with prolapse repair
	VLLP/MUCP	

be an important tool for evaluating symptomatic patients following urethral sling surgery.

In cases of persistent urinary symptoms following sling placement, urodynamics can help determine whether the sling is too tight and is causing outlet obstruction or whether the patient's symptoms may be unrelated to the outlet and involve detrusor function. Filling cystometry, pressure flow studies, and opening detrusor pressures will distinguish these patients. Opening detrusor pressures over 20–30 cm water and weak urinary flow rates with high detrusor pressures are typically suggestive of outlet obstruction. Sling removal or revision with urethrolysis may be the best option for these patients once the diagnosis is confirmed by urodynamics.

Patients with de novo urinary storage symptoms following sling placement and with urodynamic findings consistent with a normal outlet should be offered medically management before considering sling removal or revision. These patients often will respond to anticholinergics and show improvement over time. However, if symptoms persist despite initial conservative efforts, sling removal may be necessary as a treatment option. Additionally, some patients may present with recurrent SUI following sling placement. These patients may or may not demonstrate SUI on clinical exam and should be evaluated with urodynamics to better understand the dynamics involved at their bladder outlet as well as with detrusor function. Patients with low leak point pressures will likely need repeat anti-incontinence procedure, while those with detrusor overactivity and a normal outlet will need medical therapies.

5.3.3 Pelvic Organ Prolapse

Stress incontinence and POP can coexist in up to 80 % of women with pelvic floor dysfunction [15]. Many of these patients with POP have minimal or no symptoms related to urinary incontinence at the time of presentation. However, following prolapse reduction (i.e., pessary placement or following POP repair), many of these patients will demonstrate *occult stress urinary incontinence*. Therefore careful clinical and urodynamic evaluation is often necessary in all patients with POP seeking surgery. While in clinic, these patients should be examined with their prolapse reduced either with the use of a pessary or via digital reduction. These patients should be then asked to cough or bear down in order elicit any occult SUI. Patients with occult SUI seen on prolapse reduction can proceed to sling placement at the time of prolapse repair. However, patients who are unable to demonstrate occult SUI on clinical exam should proceed to urodynamics prior to surgery. Urodynamics will offer objective information regarding the bladder outlet and the relative functionality of the patient's bladder. This information is valuable for patient counseling and can help predict patient outcome following surgery.

5.4 Case Studies

5.4.1 Patient 1

5.4.1.1 History
The patient is a 65-year-old woman with a long-standing history of stress urinary incontinence s/p multiple anti-incontinence procedures. She had an MMK performed 25 years ago, followed by an RMUS 10 years ago and multiple subsequent periurethral bulking agents. She complains of stress incontinence with coughing, sneezing, exercise, and walking. She wears 6–8 pads during the day. She does void every 1–2 h, typically preemptive in order to avoid incontinence.

5.4.1.2 Physical Examination
Gen: No acute distress
CVS: RRR, no edema
Pulm: Clear to auscultation
Abd: Soft, non-tender, non-distended, and no CVA tenderness to palpation
Neuro: No focal deficits
GU: −UH, +CST, and no prolapse noted

5.4.1.3 Labwork/Other Studies
PVR—0 mL
UA—negative

5.4.1.4 UDS
See Fig. 5.3.

Findings
The filling phase demonstrated first sensation at 19 mL, first desire at 83 mL, normal desire at 156 mL, and maximum cystometric capacity at 158 mL. At cystometric capacity, there was stress incontinence noted with Valsalva, with the patient leaking approximately 69 mL. VLPP was 65 cm/H_2O, see Fig. 5.3. There was no detrusor activity noted. The voiding phase was unremarkable, demonstrating low pressure void with complete emptying. The flow was mildly reduced, likely due to volume voided.

5.4.1.5 Treatment Options
The options offered to the patient included repeat bulking agent, synthetic RMUS, and autologous fascial sling. She opted for a rectus fascial sling. Postoperatively, she went into retention and required CIC for 6 weeks. She subsequently started to void spontaneously and stopped CIC with residuals

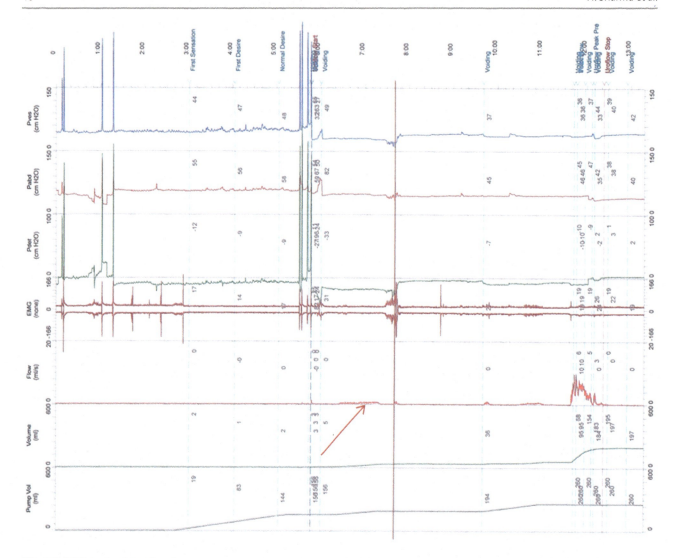

Fig. 5.3 UDS tracing for patient 1

as low as 10 mL. She remained continent with no pad usage at 1-year follow-up.

5.4.2 Patient 2

5.4.2.1 History

The patient is an 84-year-old woman with complaint of continuous incontinence. She does not void volitionally in the bathroom. She complains of continuous leakage with large-volume incontinence associated with activity. She wears 10 pull-ups per day. She has a past surgical history of vaginal hysterectomy, vault suspension, anterior/posterior repair, and urethropexy 30 years ago. She then had a synthetic RMUS 12 years ago, followed by an autologous fascial sling 5 years ago. She has been incontinent despite these procedures.

5.4.2.2 Physical Examination

Gen: No acute distress.
CVS: RRR, no edema
Pulm: Clear to auscultation
Abd: Soft, non-tender, non-distended, and no CVA tenderness to palpation
Neuro: No focal deficits
GU: −UH, +CST, and no prolapse noted

5.4.2.3 Labwork/Other Studies

PVR−0 mL
UA−negative

5 Female Stress Urinary Incontinence

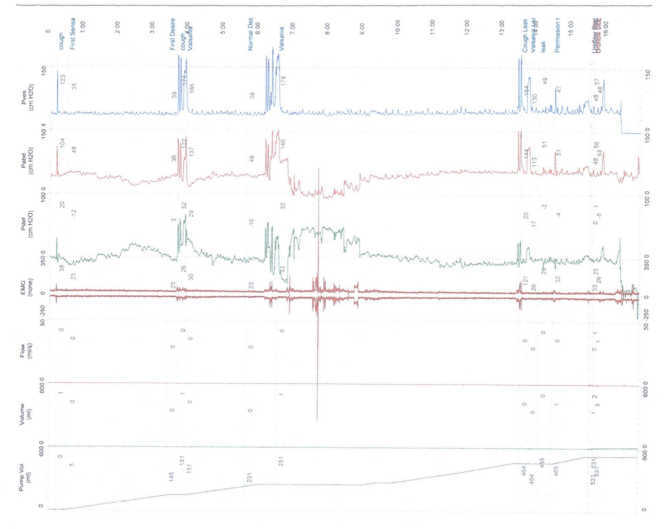

Fig. 5.4 UDS tracing for patient 2

5.4.2.4 UDS
See Fig. 5.4.

Findings
The filling phase demonstrates first sensation at 5 mL, first desire at 145 mL, and maximum cystometric capacity of 531 mL. There was no detrusor overactivity noted. There was stress urinary incontinence with LPP 113 cm/H_2O. The leak was visualized, not registered on the flow. The voiding phase was unable to be completed with the catheters in place. The noninvasive flow demonstrated normal flow with bell-shaped curve.

5.4.2.5 Treatment Options
The options offered to the patient included repeat synthetic RMUS, autologous fascial sling, or periurethral bulking agent. She opted for a periurethral bulking agent. She did well postoperatively. Six months postoperatively, she states her incontinence has improved significantly. She is able to void in the bathroom. She wears one pad per day.

5.5 Summary

Stress urinary incontinence is a diagnosis that can be made clinically in most cases based on a positive stress (cough) test. Index cases of pure SUI generally do not require urodynamics and clinicians can proceed to surgical correction of the urethra without any further testing. Complicated cases of SUI, as described in this chapter, often require urodynamic evaluation in order to determine an accurate diagnosis prior to treatment. For patients with urge-predominant mixed urinary incontinence, persistent stress incontinence despite prior anti-incontinence surgery, or pelvic organ prolapse, urodynamics is a valuable tool that can help guide management decisions prior to surgery.

References

1. Abrams P, et al. Standardization Sub-Committee of the International Continence Society: The standardization of terminology in lower urinary tract function: report from the Standardization Subcommittee of the International Continence Society. Urology. 2003;61(1):37–49.
2. Hampel C, Artibani W, Espuna Pons M, et al. Understanding the burden of stress urinary incontinence in Europe: a qualitative review of the literature. Eur Urol. 2004;46:15.
3. Van Leijsen SA, Kluivers KB, Mow BW, et al. Can preoperative urodynamic investigation be omitted in women with stress urinary incontinence? A non-inferiority randomized controlled trial. Neurourol Urodyn. 2012;31:1118–23.
4. Abram P. Urodynamics in clinical practice. In: Urodynamics. 3rd ed. London: Springer; 2006. p. 147–69 (Chapter 5).
5. Lue T, Tanagho E. Urinary incontinence. In: Smith and Tanagho's general urology. 18th ed. New York: McGraw-Hill Medical; 2013. p. 480–97 (Chapter 30).
6. Topazio L, Frey J, Iacovelli V, Perugia V, Vespasiani G, Finazzi AE. Prevalence of "complicated" stress urinary incontinence in female patients: can urodynamics provide more information in such patients? Int Urogynecol J. 2015;26(9):1333–9.
7. Blaivas J, et al. Stress incontinence in women. In: Atlas of urodynamics. 2nd ed. New York: Wiley; 2007. p. 184–5 (Chapter 15).
8. McGuire EJ. Leak point pressures. Urol Clin North Am. 1996;23:253.
9. Khullar V, Cardozo L, Dmochowski R. Mixed incontinence: current evidence and future perspectives. Neurourol Urodyn. 2010;29:618–22.
10. Nager CW, et al. A randomized trial of urodynamic testing before stress-incontinence surgery. N Engl J Med. 2012;366(21):1987–97.
11. Zyczynski H, Albo M, Goldman H, Wai C, Sirls L, Brubaker L, Norton P, Varner R, Carmel M, Kim H, Urinary Incontinence Treatment Network. Change in overactive bladder symptoms after surgery for stress urinary incontinence in women. Obstet Gynecol. 2015;126(2):423–30.
12. Palva K, Nilsson C. Prevalence of urinary urgency symptoms decreases by mid-urethral procedures for treatment of stress incontinence. Int Urogynecol J. 2011;22(10):1241–7.
13. Geller EJ, Wu JM. Changing trends in surgery for stress urinary incontinence. Curr Opin Obstet Gynecol. 2013;25(5):404–9.
14. Nitti V. Complications of midurethral slings and their management. Can Urol Assoc J. 2012;6(5 Suppl 2):S120–2.
15. Bai SW, Jeon MJ, Kim JY, Chung KA, Kim SY, Park KH. Relationship between stress urinary incontinence and pelvic organ prolapsed. Int Urogynecol J Pelvic Floor Dysfunct. 2002;13(4):256.

Male Stress Urinary Incontinence

Ricardo Palmerola and Farzeen Firoozi

6.1 Introduction

Stress urinary incontinence (SUI) is the involuntary leakage of urine with exertion or maneuvers that increase intra-abdominal pressure (coughing, sneezing, etc.) as a result of inadequate bladder outlet resistance. Stress urinary incontinence is not a common problem afflicting the general male population; however, it is encountered in urological practice and has major implications for patient's quality of life [1]. In order for a male to develop SUI, there must be dysfunction of both the internal urinary sphincter and the external urinary sphincter [2]. There are many etiologies that may cause disruption of the bladder outlet in males, the most common being iatrogenic in nature. Less commonly, SUI is encountered following pelvic trauma and disruption of the posterior urethra. Congenital neurogenic disorders (myelodysplasia) and acquired neurogenic disorders (multiple sclerosis) may also contribute to the development of SUI. Finally, unresolved urological conditions from infancy may be another risk factor for stress incontinence [3].

SUI in the male is most commonly encountered following radical prostatectomy. Nearly all patients who undergo radical surgery for prostate cancer have immediate SUI postoperatively; however, the number of patients who remain incontinent has been the subject of continued debate. Although higher rates were seen in the past, contemporary studies have reported persistent postprostatectomy incontinence ranging from 8 to 48% [4–7]. Minimally invasive and nerve sparing approaches have been purported to account for this improvement in functional outcomes; however, methods to obtain and define incontinence are heterogeneous among available studies [8, 9]. Patients undergoing surgery for benign prostatic hyperplasia may also be at risk of postoperative incontinence. The incidence of urinary incontinence following prostatectomy for benign disease has been reported to be 1–3%, while urinary incontinence following transurethral resection of prostate has been reported to be between 1 and 5% [3, 10, 11]. The incidence of urinary incontinence increases dramatically in patients who had received radiotherapy prior to their outlet procedure. In one study, 25% of patients experienced urinary incontinence in this setting (SUI, urge urinary incontinence, or both) [12].

In most men with postprostatectomy incontinence, the primary defect lies in the bladder outlet. Disruption of the sphincteric continence mechanism during surgery leads to stress incontinence in the postoperative period [13]. However, up to 40% of men with postprostatectomy incontinence have mixed incontinence, where in addition to SUI, patients may present with bladder dysfunction (overactive bladder, decreased compliance, detrusor underactivity) [14, 15]. Only 3% of patients with postprostatectomy incontinence have isolated bladder dysfunction causing their symptoms [13]. Although intrinsic urinary sphincter deficiency is the primary etiology for most postprostatectomy patients, it is imperative to elucidate all of the possible etiologies to the patient's complaint of incontinence.

6.2 Evaluation

When evaluating males with SUI, a thorough history and physical examination is critical. A focused history and comprehensive assessment of the patient's lower urinary tract symptoms should be performed in the initial evaluation.

R. Palmerola, M.D., M.S. (✉)
Department of Urology, Northwell Health System, Center for Advanced Medicine, The Arthur Smith Institute of Urology, 450 Lakeville Road, Suite M42, New Hyde Park, NY 11042, USA
e-mail: rpalmero12@northwell.edu

F. Firoozi, M.D., F.A.C.S.
Department of Urology, Northwell Health System, Center for Advanced Medicine, The Arthur Smith Institute of Urology, 450 Lakeville Road, Suite M41, New Hyde Park, NY 11042, USA
e-mail: ffiroozi@northwell.edu; ffirooziimd@gmail.com

The severity of incontinence may be graded between grade I and III based on history:

Mild (grade I) incontinence occurring with coughing and sneezing
Mild (grade II) occurring with minor exertion like walking
Severe (grade III) occurring during minimal to no exertion [9]

A subjective measure of the amount of urine lost daily, pads changed, or diapers changed daily should be documented. The presence and duration of diabetes mellitus, preceding neurological pathology, history of radiation, and pelvic trauma should be noted. If the patient underwent radical pelvic surgery, the history should focus on an assessment of urinary tract symptoms preceding surgery as well as the patient's current complaints. As mentioned earlier in the chapter, patients may present with mixed incontinence following surgery some of which may be the result of preceding bladder dysfunction or obstruction.

Assessment of quality of life can be performed using a number of validated questionnaires including I-QoL (incontinence quality of life questionnaire) and ICIQ-SF (international consultation on incontinence questionnaire short form) [9]. Quality of life information should be assessed as one study found that pad weight correlated with the degree of patient dissatisfaction with the condition [16]. Physical examination should include neurologic evaluation as well as a thorough genitourinary exam. Rectal examination should be performed to assess rectal tone, as well as the prostatic fossa in postprostatectomy patients. Stress incontinence should be demonstrated by having the patient perform Valsalva maneuvers or cough with an adequate bladder volume (typically 300 mL). A post-void residual (PVR) should be obtained, especially in patients who primarily void by Valsalva. Prior to invasive testing or treatment, urinalysis and urine culture should be obtained as urinary tract infection may aggravate urinary incontinence. A PSA should be obtained as well as routine blood chemistries and complete blood count. In diabetic patients, one may obtain an HbA1c to evaluate how well their disease is controlled. Finally, attempts should be made to gain an objective measure of the severity of urine leaked as well as functional capacity. The authors provide all patients presenting with stress incontinence a voiding diary to document the daily fluid intake, urinary frequency, and volume of urine voided as well as timing of incontinence. Although patient compliance may be a challenge, a 24-h pad test should be advised to the patient as it provides the most reliable and reproducible quantification of urine leaked daily [17].

Further studies needed to evaluate patients with male SUI include cystourethroscopy. The exam should focus on ruling out concurrent pathologies including urethral stricture disease or bladder neck contracture in patients who underwent radical prostatectomy. The integrity and tone of the urethral sphincter can be directly visualized during examination. Specifically, in patients with a history of TURP, one may appreciate disruption or absence of the verumontanum which is suggestive of external sphincter damage. Finally, one can evaluate the bladder mucosa for the presence of trabeculation and diverticula suggesting prior bladder dysfunction.

Multichannel urodynamics (UDS) is recommended to evaluate patients who are considering invasive treatment [3, 18]. UDS remains an important part of the workup of a patient with stress incontinence as it can assess bladder compliance, bladder hypersensitivity, Valsalva leak point pressure (VLPP), detrusor overactivity, detrusor contractility, and sphincteric function [15]. The use of fluoroscopy can aid in the evaluation of stress incontinence at the time of UDS. Urethral and bladder neck mobility can be assessed using fluoroscopy at the time of UDS, and it can demonstrate contrast leakage alongside the catheter. In patients with concomitant bladder dysfunction, or mixed urinary incontinence, UDS findings help guide clinicians in selecting the best treatment.

For example, the decision to undergo artificial urethral sphincter (AUS) rather than bulbourethral sling placement may be made based on the status of bladder contractility during UDS [15]. Recent studies have questioned the utility of UDS in predicting outcomes for patients requiring surgical management of stress incontinence. The authors showed that adverse findings on urodynamics including detrusor overactivity, low cystometric capacity, low abdominal leak point pressure, low Q_{max}, and poor bladder contractility did not adversely affect outcomes of continence procedures [19, 20]. Despite the potential risk of damage to the upper urinary tract, one author suggested that poor compliance in otherwise neurologically intact patients may be due to the urinary incontinence itself. Improvement of stress incontinence may recover bladder elasticity by restoring normal bladder cycling [21]. Despite this new evidence, ICS guidelines support the use of multichannel urodynamics prior to invasive treatment.

6.3 Management

The treatment options for men with stress incontinence are primarily surgical. In men with postprostatectomy incontinence, nonoperative options within 1 year of surgery include pelvic floor muscle training or Kegel exercises. Other nonoperative interventions include biofeedback therapy and electrical stimulation of the pudendal nerve; however, clinical efficacy has been limited for these approaches [9, 22]. In fact, most large centers typically have a postprostatectomy rehabilitation program that addresses incontinence issues in the first year after surgery for prostate cancer.

Once conservative management has been exhausted, surgical intervention may be considered. Surgical options are limited to periurethral bulking agents, bulbourethral slings, and AUS. Periurethral bulking agents represent the least invasive approach to surgical intervention; however, long-term success and durability are modest. One randomized study comparing AUS to Macroplastique™ (Cogentix Medical, Minnetonka, MN, USA) injections showed no statistically significant difference in outcomes in patients with minimal incontinence (<100 g pad weight per day) [23]. Although multiple procedures may be necessary in some patients, these results suggest that Macroplastique injections may be a reasonable option for patients with mild stress urinary incontinence. The male sling has emerged as an efficacious surgical option for men with stress incontinence. Several procedures have been described including a transobturator bulbourethral sling (AdVance™, Boston Scientific, Marlborough, MA, USA), a combined retropubic and transobturator (Virtue™, Coloplast Corp., Minneapolis, MN, USA), and the bone-anchored perineal sling (InVance™, Boston Scientific, Marlborough, MA, USA) [24–28]. Finally, the AUS serves as the gold standard for postprostatectomy stress incontinence. The device has also been used successfully in appropriately selected cases including pediatric patients with myelodysplasia, neurogenic bladder, and incontinence following radical cystoprostatectomy and creation of orthotopic neobladder [3].

6.4 Case Studies

6.4.1 Patient 1

6.4.1.1 History

This patient is a 57-year-old gentleman with a chief complaint of urinary incontinence that began immediately following a robotic radical prostatectomy 3 years prior to referral. In the immediate postoperative period, he experienced urine leakage with cough and moderate levels of activity. Over time he developed irritative lower urinary tract symptoms (LUTS) consisting of urinary urgency and diurnal urinary frequency. He denied any obstructive LUTS, recent urinary tract infection, or hematuria. In the immediate postoperative period, he was instructed to perform Kegel exercises, which he performed on occasion and did not improve his symptoms. At the time of referral, he was using two pads daily, with the degree of saturation varying daily. At night he used a pad; however, it was typically dry. On follow-up, he completed a voiding diary as well as a 24-h pad test, which showed that his total pad weight was 105 g. His past medical history was remarkable for hypertension and localized prostate cancer.

6.4.1.2 Physical Examination

General: no acute distress, appearing his stated age.
Psychologic: no signs of depression.
Neurologic: normal gait and sensory examination.
Cardiovascular: no labored breathing or extremity edema.
Abdomen: soft, nontender, and nondistended.
Genitourinary: no costovertebral tenderness, circumcised phallus with no lesions, bilaterally descended testes with no masses, and no inguinal hernias bilaterally. Rectal exam was notable for normal sphincter tone and an empty prostatic fossa. He was asked to perform a Valsalva maneuver as well as cough which provoked visible urine loss.

6.4.1.3 Labwork/Other Studies

UA was within normal limits.
Urine culture was negative.
PSA was undetectable.
PVR 0 mL.
Cystourethroscopy performed in the office, which revealed no urethral strictures, bladder neck contractures, or mucosal abnormalities in the bladder. Able to contract EUS.

6.4.1.4 UDS

See Fig. 6.1.

Findings

Prior to commencing the procedure, the patient voided 461 mL, and on uroflowmetry, he achieved a Q_{max} of 44 mL/s and a Q_{avg} of 20 mL/s.

Filling Phase
- First desire 148 mL.
- No DO. There are several negative deflections in P_{det} tracing. These negative tracings are likely secondary to rectal contractions and are not considered an abnormal finding (a on Fig. 6.1).
- Normal desire 352 mL.
- Cystometric capacity was 651 mL.
- The patient was asked to perform Valsalva maneuvers during this examination, which did not recreate his symptoms. The points at which he performed Valsalva are characterized by the sharp rise in intra-abdominal, intravesical pressure and flat P_{det} tracing (b on Fig. 6.1). The EMG tracing correlates with the Valsalva maneuvers suggesting the presence of sphincteric activity (c on Fig. 6.1). Bladder compliance was normal and P_{det} at capacity was 9 cm/H_2O. After catheter was removed, with Valsalva, the patient did have incontinence.

Voiding Phase
- Q_{max} was 35 mL/s and average flow was 17 mL/s.
- At p_{Det}, Q_{max} was 21 cm/H_2O.
- Shape of the flow curve appears to be a normal bell curve.
- Total voided volume was 720 mL and PVR was 0 mL.

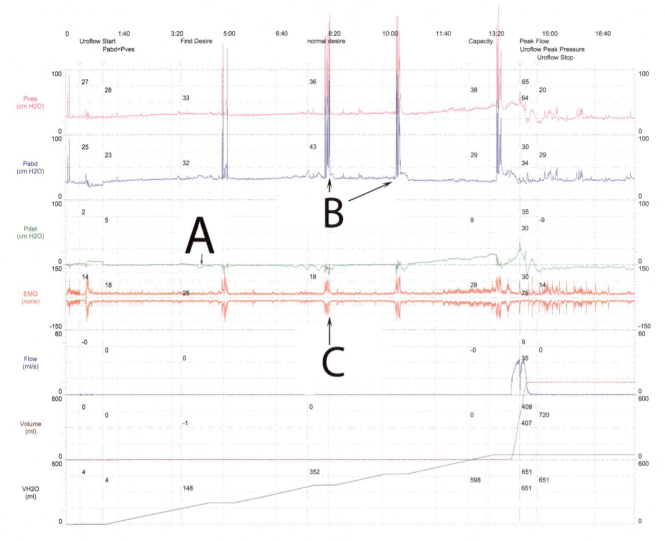

Fig. 6.1 Patient 1: urodynamics tracing

In summary this patient's UDS showed that he has normal bladder sensation, a normal bladder capacity, and normal compliance. Urodynamic stress incontinence was not demonstrated in the study; however, it had been demonstrated in physical exam. This can occur during UDS in postprostatectomy patients who may have decreased urethral compliance in addition to the urethral catheter used during the exam. This can be explained in this patient by the discrepancy in his preprocedure uroflowmetry ($Q_{max} = 44$ mL/s) and his voiding phase during UDS ($Q_{max} = 35$ mL/s). He does demonstrate a low detrusor pressure at Q_{max}; however, this does not reflect a poorly contractile bladder as the urethral resistance may be diminished in a patient with stress incontinence secondary to intrinsic sphincter deficiency.

6.4.1.5 Treatment Options
– Penile clamping device
– Periurethral bulking agents
– Male sling
– AUS

Being that he expressed a significant amount of distress over his symptoms, male sling and AUS were offered as the best option for success. In this patient with mild to moderate stress incontinence, no history of radiation, demonstrable stress incontinence on exam, and adequate bladder contractility, he was a good candidate for either procedure. When given the option, most patients with postprostatectomy incontinence choose to undergo placement of male sling to avoid a mechanical device [24]. He elected to undergo placement of an AdVance™ transobturator sling. Postoperatively, he passed his void trial and his PVR was 0 mL. He has remained continent 2 years postoperatively, does not use pads, and has not undergone secondary procedures.

6.4.2 Patient 2

6.4.2.1 History

This patient is a 65-year-old gentleman with a chief complaint of urinary incontinence following a radical prostatectomy 2 years prior to referral. His symptoms occurred exclusively when he coughed, sneezed, lifted heavy objects, or performed any moderate amount of activity. At night he used a safety napkin and he used three napkins on a daily basis (only used napkins rather than pads). He had no other lower urinary tract symptoms and past medical history was significant for a herniated lumbar disk. Prior to referral, he had tried Kegel exercises and utilized a penile clamp; however, he had unsatisfactory results with both. On follow-up, he completed 1 day of a voiding diary notable for a morning void of 350 mL and did not find time to perform a 24-h pad test.

6.4.2.2 Physical Examination

General: no acute distress, appearing his stated age.
Psychologic: no signs of depression.
Neurologic: normal gait and sensory examination.
Cardiovascular: no labored breathing or extremity edema.
Abdomen: soft, nontender, nondistended, well-healed incision.
Genitourinary: napkin with urine spotting, a circumcised phallus without lesions or plaques. The testes were descended bilaterally, firm, nontender, and without masses, and there were no inguinal hernias bilaterally. Digital rectal exam revealed normal sphincter tone and an empty prostatic fossa. He was asked to perform a Valsalva maneuver and as a result he leaked several drops of urine.

6.4.2.3 Labwork/Other Studies

- PSA was undetectable.
- UA and urine culture negative.
- PVR 0 mL.
- Cystourethroscopy was performed, notable for the absence of urethral stricture, bladder neck contracture, and no abnormalities were noted along the bladder mucosa. Able to contract EUS.

6.4.2.4 UDS

See Fig. 6.2.

Findings

The patient underwent urodynamics to continue his evaluation; however, throughout the exam he was quite uncomfortable and did not tolerate bladder filling.

Filling Phase

- First sensation 100 mL.
- First desire to void was noted at 207 mL.
- Normal desire to void occurred at 224 mL.
- DO noted.
- SUI (SUI noted without catheter on initial exam). No UUI noted.
- Cystometric capacity was 247 mL.

Voiding Phase

During the voiding phase, a Q_{max} of 17 mL/s was obtained with a P_{det} of 18 cm/H$_2$O at Q_{max}. There was a normal bell curve during the voiding phase, and the patient's PVR was 14 mL. It is also important to note the absence of high abdominal pressures during the voiding phase, suggesting the patient does not normally perform a Valsalva maneuver to void.

In summary this patient's UDS demonstrated normal compliance, detrusor overactivity, and reduced bladder capacity. The utility of a voiding diary becomes evident in this patient's case. His first morning void was approximately 375 mL, suggesting that functional capacity was not represented in the examination (likely from discomfort). Additionally, detrusor overactivity was noted during the examination although he did not complain of urinary urgency and frequency. The presence of detrusor overactivity is not unusual in postprostatectomy patients and is reported to be as high as 40 % of postprostatectomy patients during UDS [13, 15].

6.4.2.5 Treatment Options

- Penile clamping device
- Periurethral bulking agents
- Male sling
- AUS

This patient elected to undergo placement of an AdVance™ male sling. Postoperatively he had complete resolution of his stress incontinence and did not require the use of pads. He was able to void without difficulty and his PVR was 0 mm. Unfortunately, the patient presented after 2 years with recurrent stress incontinence for which he resumed using sanitary pads. He also complained of increased urinary frequency (voiding up to 15 times daily), urinary urgency, and nocturia. On his voiding diary, it was noted he was drinking approximately 1 L of herbal tea and coffee in addition to water and 3–4 glasses of wine after dinner. After behavioral modification including fluid restriction, caffeine restriction, and decreasing alcohol consumption, his OAB symptoms improved. He did continue to experience stress incontinence and he underwent videourodynamics as part of his new evaluation.

6.4.2.6 UDS

See Fig. 6.3.

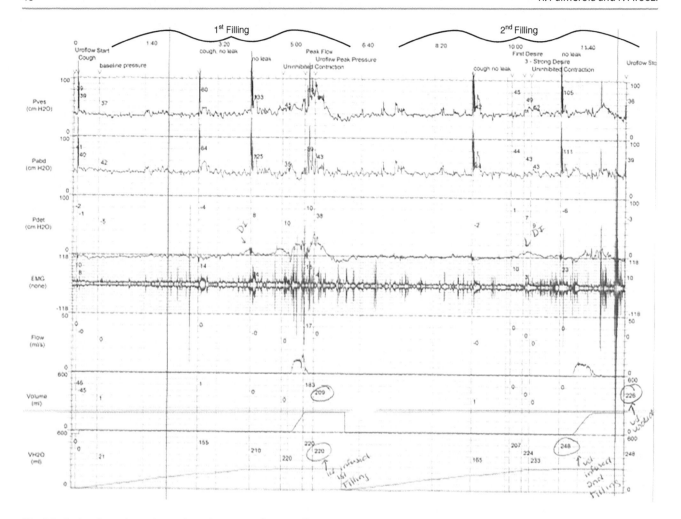

Fig. 6.2 Patient 2: urodynamics tracing prior to transobturator sling

Filling Phase
- First sensation was noted at 92 mL.
- First desire at 147 mL.
- Normal desire at 207 mL.
- Cystometric capacity at 313 mL.
- No DO noted.
- Bladder compliance was normal.
- VLPP was measured at 90 cm/H_2O (volume 255 mL), as this was the lowest intravesical pressure where he leaked.

Voiding Phase
- Q_{max} was 17 mL/s.
- P_{det} at Q_{max} = 39 cm/H_2O.
- Total voided volume was 246 mL and PVR was 66 mL. On fluoroscopy his bladder had a normal contour and leakage was noted as contrast passed alongside the catheter. As he voided there was funneling of the bladder neck and kinking at the location of the sling.

In summary, the second UDS showed resolution of his detrusor overactivity seen on his prior study, stress incontinence with an abdominal leak point pressure of 90 cm/H_2O, and a nonobstructed bladder outlet (bladder outlet index = 5).

6.4.2.7 Treatment Options
- Periurethral bulking agent
- Repeat male sling
- AUS

For patients who have failed surgical management with a male sling and continue to have continued stress incontinence, a repeat urodynamics is warranted. One needs to reassess bladder compliance, detrusor function, and rule out obstruction. Prior to subjecting the patient to a second procedure, further investigation is warranted to treat any underlying etiology to mixed urinary incontinence. Furthermore, videourodynamics (Fig. 6.4a,b) can be utilized to visualize the degree of mobility in the proximal urethra, sling

6 Male Stress Urinary Incontinence

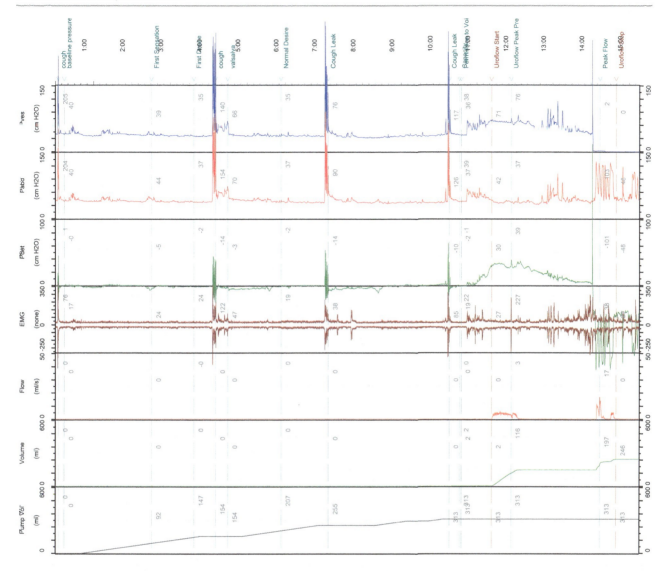

Fig. 6.3 Patient 2: urodynamics tracing after treatment failure with transobturator sling

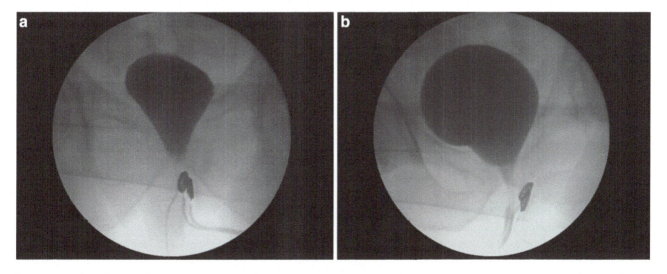

Fig. 6.4 (**a**, **b**) Fluoroscopic images for patient 2 captured during videourodynamics prior to undergoing implantation of artificial urinary sphincter. Both images capture funneling of the bladder neck and urethral kinking likely caused by the transobturator sling

placement, and examine the contour of the bladder. After the appropriate workup is obtained, patients who fail therapy with a male sling can be considered for placement of an AUS. Several studies have reported promising outcomes and patient satisfaction after a failed male sling [29, 30].

The patient underwent placement of AUS and postoperatively had resolution of his stress incontinence after activating the device. He has continued to remain fully continent, requiring no pads up to 1 year postoperatively at last follow-up.

6.4.3 Patient 3

6.4.3.1 History

This patient is a 77-year-old gentleman presenting for evaluation of urinary incontinence of 1 year. His past urologic history is significant for prostate cancer treated with brachytherapy 13 years ago. One year prior to current evaluation, he began experiencing obstructive voiding symptoms and subsequently underwent a Greenlight™ (American Medical Systems, Minnetonka, MN, USA) laser photovaporization of the prostate (PVP). Postoperatively he developed severe incontinence, consisting of continuous leakage, exacerbated by light activity and typically high in volume. Although he was voiding volitionally, the volume actually voided was typically lower than the preoperative state. On average he was using 6–8 pads daily and most nights would need at least one pad change. He had no other voiding symptoms and denied gross hematuria. In addition to prostate cancer, he had a history of diabetes mellitus, coronary artery disease, and hyperlipidemia. He had undergone a CABG 11 years prior and was currently on antiplatelet therapy consisting of aspirin and clopidogrel. Prior to his follow-up appointment, he completed a 3-day voiding diary significant for low fluid intake and low voided volumes. His 24 h pad weight was over 600 g.

6.4.3.2 Physical Examination

General: no acute distress, appearing his stated age.
Psychologic: no signs of depression.
Neurologic: normal gait and sensory examination.
Cardiovascular: no labored breathing or extremity edema.
Abdomen: soft, nontender, and nondistended.
Genitourinary: circumcised phallus without lesions or plaques, testes descended bilaterally, and approximately 25 mL in volume. The epididymides were flat bilaterally and no inguinal hernias were present bilaterally. On digital rectal examination, he had normal rectal tone and no rectal masses, and the prostate was approximately 45 cm^3, firm, and flat consistent with prior radiation therapy. When asked to perform a Valsalva maneuver, he leaked significantly.

6.4.3.3 Labwork/Other Studies

- PSA which was unchanged from nadir.
- Urinalysis was obtained revealing microscopic hematuria, presence of leukocyte esterase and nitrites. Urine culture was positive for multiple organisms including *E. coli* and *Enterococcus faecalis*. He received a full course of antibiotics and subsequent negative urine culture prior to undergoing flexible cystoscopy. Of note, incontinence did not change after treatment.
- Cystoscopy was significant for bladder wall trabeculation; a small diverticulum in the posterior wall of the bladder, friable prostatic tissue, and the verumontanum could not be clearly identified. There were no urethral strictures or mucosal abnormalities of the bladder.

6.4.3.4 UDS

See Fig. 6.5.

Findings

Filling Phase

- First sensation occurred at 191 mL.
- Normal desire to void occurred at 220 mL.
- DO noted (a on Fig. 6.5). Concomitantly, the patient leaked 50 mL around the catheter, which was depicted by the technician and generated enough flow to appear on the flow tracing (b on Fig. 6.5).
- Detrusor leak point pressure was measured at 33 cm/H$_2$O, as this was the pressure he began leaking in the absence of increased abdominal pressure.
- Synergic EMG response to detrusor overactivity. After the detrusor instability is resolved, bladder filling was resumed, and he reached a cystometric capacity of 279 mL, with a detrusor pressure of 4 cm/H$_2$O. When he was asked to perform a Valsalva during the exam, stress incontinence was not demonstrated (c on Fig. 6.5).

Voiding Phase

The voiding phase of this study was limited by patient discomfort as he was trying to void with the catheter in place.

- Q_{max} was 4.9 mL/s.
- P_{det} at Q_{max} was 41 cm/H$_2$O.
- Only voided 83 mL with the urethral catheter in place, and after it was removed, he voided 221 mL with a Q_{max} of 7 mL/s.

In summary, his UDS showed diminished bladder sensation, reduced bladder capacity, and a detrusor leak point pressure of 33 cm/H$_2$O. Urodynamics in this patient was an important intervention, as it helped discover concurrent voiding dysfunction. Although the patient did not complain

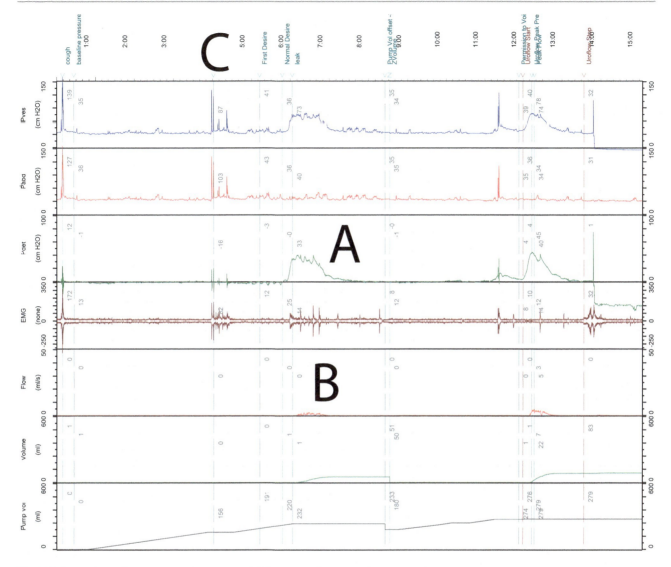

Fig. 6.5 Patient 3: urodynamics tracing prior to artificial urinary sphincter implantation

of urgency or urge incontinence at the time of referral, this was only achieved with a volume of 232 mL. With the severity of his incontinence, he may have not amounted sufficient volumes to experience detrusor overactivity. Given the information gained from this exam, one can address multiple aspects of his voiding dysfunction.

6.4.3.5 Treatment Options

In this patient with stress predominant urinary incontinence, detrusor overactivity, and a complex medical history, there are several considerations that must be taken when formulating a treatment plan. Although this patient's presentation is complex, a multimodal approach may successfully address his voiding dysfunction. In patients with brachytherapy, there is a small risk of experiencing urinary incontinence. Unfortunately these patients are also at risk for urinary retention as well as irritative voiding symptoms including urgency.

For those patients managed with transurethral resection of prostate (TURP), the risk of becoming incontinent increases dramatically [12]. Although the patient did not undergo TURP, patients undergoing PVP have a similar risk of permanent incontinence [3]. Surgical management for stress incontinence following procedures for bladder outlet obstruction is best defined for AUS. Given the patient's presentation, he would not be a candidate for a male sling owing primarily to the severity of incontinence and his prior history of radiotherapy. AUS has become the gold standard for the management of lame stress incontinence, primarily in patients with postprostatectomy incontinence for malignant and benign disease [30]. Multiple studies have demonstrated a satisfactory and durable outcome for incontinence as well as patient satisfaction [31, 32]. The risk of reoperation is one that must be addressed prior to intervention as it can approach rates as high as 29%, secondary to mechanical failure, erosion, or postoperative infection [31]. The patient's history of radiation does not preclude him from surgical management as contemporary studies have shown similar outcomes to nonradiated patients [30]. Additionally, unfavorable UDS features, including detrusor overactivity, have been reported to have no detrimental effects on continence postimplantation [20].

The patient was counseled on his medical and surgical options and was initiated on anticholinergic therapy, which did significantly improve his OAB symptoms, and he was able to demonstrate larger voided volumes based on voiding diary. Initially he decided to forgo surgical management and used a penile clamp to maintain continence. After 1 year, he returned for follow-up and underwent placement of an AUS. Postoperatively, he began cycling his device and was using one pad daily as a safety pad, which he is satisfied with using.

6.5 Summary

Urinary incontinence in males is less prevalent than the disease in female counterparts. Stress incontinence in males can be detrimental to quality of life and may coexist with other voiding symptoms. Although there are several etiologies for male stress incontinence, the most common occurs after radical prostatectomy. As in most patients with male stress incontinence, the etiology may be obtained from clinical exam; however, the use of urodynamics plays an important role prior to subjecting the patient to invasive treatment. The data obtained from urodynamics may assist in treatment planning by assessing the functional capacity of the bladder and detecting bladder dysfunction. Although recent data suggest that urodynamics may not be necessary, expert opinion suggests that it remains a valuable tool prior to surgical management of male stress incontinence.

References

1. Markland AD, Richter HE, Fwu CW, Eggers P, Kusek JW. Prevalence and trends of urinary incontinence in adults in the United States, 2001 to 2008. J Urol. 2011;186(2):589–93.
2. Wessels H, Peterson AC. Surgical procedures for sphincteric incontinence in the male: the artificial genitourinary sphincter and perineal sling procedures. In: Wein AJ, Kavoussi LR, Novick AC, Partin AW, Peters CA, editors. Campbell-Walsh urology. 10th ed. Philadelphia: Saunders; 2010. p. 2290–306.
3. Herschorn S, Bruschini H, Comiter C, Goldman HB, Grise P, Hanus T, et al. Surgical treatment of urinary incontinence in men. In: Abrams P, Cardozo L, Khoury S, Wein A, editors. Incontinence. 5th ed. Bristol: International Consultation on Urologic Diseases; 2013. p. 1229–305.
4. Ficarra V, Borghesi M, Suardi N, Naeyer GD, Novara G, Schatteman P, et al. Long term evaluation of survival, continence and potency (SCP) outcomes after robot-assisted radical prostatectomy (RARP). BJU Int. 2013;112(3):338–45.
5. Boorjian SA, Eastham JA, Graefen M, Guillonneau B, Karnes RJ, Moul JW, et al. A critical analysis of the long-term impact of radical prostatectomy on cancer control and function outcomes. Eur Urol. 2012;61(4):664–75.
6. Chughtai B, Sedrakyan A, Isaacs AJ, Mao J, Lee R, Te A, et al. National study of utilization of male incontinence procedures. Neurourol Urodyn. 2016;35(1):74–80.
7. Kao TC, Cruess DF, Garner D, Foley J, Seay T, Friedrichs P, et al. Multicenter patient self-reporting questionnaire on impotence, incontinence, and stricture after radical prostatectomy. J Urol. 2000;163(3):858–64.
8. Tewari AK, Ali A, Metgud S, Theckumparampil N, Srivastava A, Khani F, et al. Functional outcomes following robotic prostatectomy using athermal, traction free risk-stratified grades of nerve sparing. World J Urol. 2013;31(3):471–80.
9. Bauer RM, Roosen A. Evaluation and treatment of postprostatectomy incontinence. AUA update series. Vol. 31;2012. p. 368–395. (Lesson 39).
10. Winters JC. Male slings in the treatment of sphincteric incompetence. Urol Clin North Am. 2011;38(1):73–81, vi–vii.
11. Foote J, Yun S, Leach GE. Postprostatectomy incontinence. Pathophysiology, evaluation, and management. Urol Clin North Am. 1991;18(2):229–41.
12. Mock S, Leapman M, Stock RG, Hall SJ, Stone NN. Risk of urinary incontinence following post-brachytherapy transurethral resection of the prostate and correlation with clinical and treatment parameters. J Urol. 2013;190(5):1805–10.
13. Groutz A, Blaivas JG, Chaikin DC, Weiss JP, Verhaaren M. The pathophysiology of post-radical prostatectomy incontinence: a clinical and video urodynamic study. J Urol. 2000;163(6):1767–70.
14. Winters JC, Appell RA, Rackley RR. Urodynamic findings in postprostatectomy incontinence. Neurourol Urodyn. 1998;17(5):493–8.
15. Jura YH, Comiter CV. Urodynamics for postprostatectomy incontinence: when are they helpful and how do we use them? Urol Clin North Am. 2014;41(3):419–27, viii.
16. Nitti VW, Mourtzinos A, Brucker BM. Correlation of patient perception of pad use with objective degree of incontinence measured by pad test in men with post-prostatectomy incontinence: the SUFU pad test study. J Urol. 2014;192(3):836–42.
17. Dylewski DA, Jamison MG, Borawski KM, Sherman ND, Amundsen CL, Webster GD. A statistical comparison of pad numbers versus pad weights in the quantification of urinary incontinence. Neurourol Urodyn. 2007;26(1):3–7.
18. Winters JC, Dmochowski RR, Goldman HB, Herndon CD, Kobashi KC, Kraus SR, et al. Urodynamic studies in adults: AUA/SUFU guideline. J Urol. 2012;188(6 Suppl):2464–72.
19. Ballert KN, Nitti VW. Association between detrusor overactivity and postoperative outcomes in patients undergoing male bone anchored perineal sling. J Urol. 2010;183(2):641–5.
20. Lai HH, Hsu EI, Boone TB. Urodynamic testing in evaluation of postradical prostatectomy incontinence before artificial urinary sphincter implantation. Urology. 2009;73(6):1264–9.
21. Mcguire EJ. Editorial comment on collagen injection therapy for post-radical retropubic prostatectomy incontinence: role of Valsalva leak point pressure. J Urol. 1997;158(6):2136.
22. Young DB, Omeis BN, Kraus SR. The role of pelvic floor rehabilitation therapy for post-prostatectomy incontinence. AUA update series. Vol. 31;2012. p. 398–407. (Lesson 40).
23. Imamoglu MA, Tuygun C, Bakirtas H, Yigitbasi O, Kiper A. The comparison of artificial urinary sphincter implantation and endourethral macroplastique injection for the treatment of post-prostatectomy incontinence. Eur Urol. 2005;47(2):209–13.
24. Kumar A, Litt ER, Ballert KN, Nitti VW. Artificial urinary sphincter versus male sling for post-prostatectomy incontinence—what do patients choose? J Urol. 2009;181(3):1231–5.

25. Davies TO, Bepple JL, McCammon KA. Urodynamic changes and initial results of the AdVance male sling. Urology. 2009;74(2):354–7.
26. Migliari R, Pistolesi D, Leone P, Viola D, Trovarelli S. Male bulbourethral sling after radical prostatectomy: intermediate outcomes at 2 to 4-year followup. J Urol. 2006;176(5):2114–8.
27. Fischer MC, Huckabay C, Nitti VW. The male perineal sling: assessment and prediction of outcome. J Urol. 2007;177(4):1414–8.
28. Li H, Gill BC, Nowacki AS, Montague DK, Angermeier KW, Wood HM, et al. Therapeutic durability of the male transobturator sling: midterm patient reported outcomes. J Urol. 2012;187(4):1331–5.
29. Fisher MB, Aggarwal N, Vuruskan H, Singla AK. Efficacy of artificial urinary sphincter implantation after failed bone-anchored male sling for postprostatectomy incontinence. Urology. 2007;70(5):942–4.
30. James MH, McCammon KA. Artificial urinary sphincter for postprostatectomy incontinence: a review. Int J Urol. 2014;21(6):536–43.
31. Gousse AE, Madjar S, Lambert MM, Fishman IJ. Artificial urinary sphincter for post-radical prostatectomy urinary incontinence. long-term subjective results. J Urol. 2001;166(5):1755–8.
32. Montague DK, Angermeier KW, Paolone DR. Long-term continence and patient satisfaction after artificial sphincter implantation for urinary incontinence after prostatectomy. J Urol. 2001;166(2):547–9.

Bladder Outlet Obstruction: Male Non-neurogenic

Christopher Hartman and David Y. Chan

7.1 Introduction

Benign prostatic hyperplasia (BPH) is one of the most common conditions in the aging male population [1]. As compared to 8% of men aged 31–40 who are diagnosed with BPH, nearly 50% of men in their sixth decade of life receive this diagnosis. Additionally, over 80% of men aged 80 or older have been diagnosed with BPH [2]. Other less common causes of bladder outlet obstruction (BOO) in male patients include urethral strictures due to trauma or infection, bladder tumors, prostate cancer, and bladder stones.

BPH develops as a hyperplasia of both stromal and epithelial components of the transition zone of the prostate. This results in large, relatively discrete, benign nodules that, with sufficient growth, may impinge on the urethral lumen and cause obstruction to the flow of urine [3]. This obstruction produces the characteristic lower urinary tract symptoms (LUTS), such as a weak urinary stream, post-void dribbling, hesitancy, intermittency, frequency, and nocturia, that are often seen in men with BPH [4].

Under the influence of testosterone, the natural history of BPH is progression. Hyperplastic nodules will continue to enlarge, producing a greater degree of obstruction over time [5]. This may lead to secondary complications of BPH, including urinary tract infections, bladder stones, detrusor hypertrophy, urinary retention, the formation of bladder diverticula, and renal deterioration due to obstructive uropathy. Early intervention may prevent development of adverse secondary effects of BPH.

Risks for BOO secondary to urethral strictures include sexually transmitted diseases (STDs), such as gonococcal and chlamydial urethritis, blunt and penetrating pelvic trauma, and previous transurethral procedures [6–8]. Whereas patients with urethral strictures secondary to STDs often report progressively worsening difficulty with voiding and a slow urinary stream, patients with urethral strictures secondary to pelvic trauma usually have a discrete inciting event and may have associated pelvic fractures or other pelvic injuries. These patients typically have a urethral disruption resulting in partial or complete obliteration of the urethral lumen. Patients who present with BOO secondary to bladder stones or lower urinary tract malignancy may report hematuria or irritative voiding symptoms in addition to obstructive voiding symptoms. It is important to rule out obstruction from other causes in patients who present with bladder stones, as these patients often have concomitant BOO from other causes such as BPH.

Numerous risk factors for the development of BPH have been proposed. The Massachusetts Male Aging Study found that the use of a beta-blocker (OR 1.8), heart disease (OR 2.1), and elevated-free PSA levels (OR 4.4) all conferred increased odds of being diagnosed with BPH. In the same study, researchers found that cigarette smoking (OR 0.5) and a higher level of physical activity each decreased the odds of being diagnosed with BPH [9]. While the Massachusetts Male Aging Study did not demonstrate a significant correlation with body mass index or the presence of diabetes, other studies have demonstrated that obesity, elevated fasting glucose levels, and a diagnosis of diabetes or metabolic syndrome may confer an increased risk of BPH [10–12].

Mixed results have also been reported for the effect of race on benign prostatic enlargement. Numerous studies have demonstrated that men of Asian descent may have a lower risk of being diagnosed with BPH, as well as a lower risk of clinically significant BPH requiring surgery [13, 14]. These studies additionally showed that the risk of BPH in black and white men is similar.

In men for whom a diagnosis of BOO is suspected, a thorough history should be obtained. This should include a history of obstructive voiding symptoms, the presence of diabetes, symptoms suggestive of neurologic disease, a

---

C. Hartman, M.D. (✉) • D.Y. Chan, M.D.
Department of Urology, Hofstra North Shore—LIJ, The Smith Institute for Urology, 450 Lakeville Rd, Suite M42, New Hyde Park, NY 11042, USA
e-mail: chartman@nshs.edu; dchan@nshs.edu

history of pelvic trauma or sexually transmitted diseases, and a family history of prostate cancer or BPH. The American Urologic Association (AUA) symptom score may be used to assess the severity of a patient's symptoms. Physical exam should be performed, paying particular attention to the neurologic exam, which could offer insight into potential bladder hypocontractility, and a digital rectal exam to assess prostate size and contour. Laboratory evaluation may include urinalysis. Creatinine should be obtained if there is concern for renal deterioration [15]. PSA testing may also be warranted if there is concern for occult prostate malignancy and screening is indicated.

Whereas previously, there were limited options for the management of patients presenting with BPH, numerous recent medical and surgical advancements in the treatment of this disease have allowed urologists to tailor treatment individually to patients based on the size of the gland, their comorbidities, and wishes. Medical therapy in the form of alpha-blockers and 5-alpha-reductase inhibitors has been shown to be superior to placebo, both alone and in combination, in reducing AUA symptom score, urinary retention, renal insufficiency, urinary tract infections, and the need for invasive therapy [16]. Minor, office-based surgical procedures such as transurethral microwave therapy and transurethral prostatic lifts can now be performed, as well as various surgical procedures such as transurethral resection of the prostate, photovaporization of the prostate, laser enucleation of the prostate, and simple prostatectomy. Similarly, surgical procedures for urethral strictures may include urethral dilation, internal urethrotomy, and urethroplasty. These procedures should all be tailored to each individual patient.

While urodynamic testing is not routinely recommended for the male patient presenting with presumed BOO, numerous circumstances warrant its inclusion when evaluating these patients. In patients with global neurological deficits, such as those with spinal cord injuries, Parkinson's disease, multiple sclerosis, cerebrovascular accidents, and neuromuscular diseases, urodynamic testing may aid in differentiating impaired contractility or sphincteric dysfunction from BOO. In patients younger than 50 years of age who present with LUTS suggestive of BOO, urodynamic testing should also be considered due to the high incidence of nonobstructive etiologies in this population [17]. Additionally, in patients who have undergone treatment for BOO and have failed, urodynamic testing should be employed to determine whether BOO still exists or underlying bladder decompensation is also present. The American Urological Association advises that urodynamic testing should be considered optional in men presenting with LUTS [18].

Urodynamic testing in patients with BOO usually demonstrates a number of characteristic findings. The hallmark of BOO is low flow (low Q_{max}) and high detrusor pressure during the voiding phase of UDS. This has been demonstrated in a number of studies, and obstruction is typically considered when Q_{max} is less than 15 mL/s [19, 20]. It has previously been demonstrated that obstruction is present in 90% of men with a $Q_{max} < 10$ mL/s [20]. Low flow rates may also be observed in disorders of poor bladder contractility, and UDS is uniquely positioned to help define normal compared to poor contractility in these men. It is important to note, however, that random variations in flow rate and detrusor pressure may be observed in single patients on pressure-flow urodynamic testing. Abrams et al. demonstrated that random variations of approximately 9–14 cm H_2O in bladder pressure measurements and 0.4–2 mL/s variations in maximum flow rate occur when performing multiple tests of urodynamics in the same patient [21].

Using Q_{max} and P_{det} at Q_{max}, one can calculate a bladder outlet obstruction index (BOOI), which, as defined by Abrams et al., may predict obstruction in men. Using the formula: $BOOI = P_{det}Q_{max} - 2(Q_{max})$, men with a BOOI greater than 40 are considered to be obstructed, while those with a BOOI less than 20 are considered to be unobstructed. Between 20 and 40, obstruction is considered to be equivocal [22].

Though BOO is often known for its effects on voiding, numerous abnormalities of bladder storage are observed as well and can be demonstrated on urodynamic testing. This is hypothesized to be the result of changes in bladder structure as a result of chronic obstruction and requirements for increased pressure in patients with BOO. Specifically on UDS, detrusor overactivity (DO) and impaired bladder compliance have been demonstrated. Studies have shown that approximately two thirds of men with BOO have DO [23, 24], that the severity of DO may be correlated to the severity of BOO [24], and, that, after intervention for BOO, DO improves or resolves in up to 67% of patients [23]. Similarly, decreased bladder compliance has also been shown to be associated with BOO and improves with treatment of BOO [25].

7.2 Case Studies

7.2.1 Patient 1

7.2.1.1 History

The patient is an 81-year-old man with mild Parkinson's disease presented with a long history of straining to void a weak urinary stream, post-void dribbling, and the feeling of incomplete bladder emptying. He had previously been managed successfully for a number of years with daily tamsulosin. Recently, however, he developed urinary retention with a failure to void for 3 days and was admitted to the hospital with acute kidney injury. He was started on finasteride at this time and over the course of the next month was given three separate trials of spontaneous voiding. After failing to void with each of these trials, he was started on a regimen of clean intermittent catheterization (CIC) every 8 h. Though he tolerated this regimen well, he developed a urinary tract infection (UTI) and was again admitted to the hospital with sepsis secondary to his UTI. After resolution of this acute episode, he was discharged from the hospital with follow-up for his urinary retention.

7.2.1.2 Physical Examination

General: no acute distress, appearing his stated age.
Psychologic: no signs of depression.
Neurologic: resting tremor with bradykinesia.
Cardiovascular: no labored breathing or extremity edema.
Abdomen: soft, nontender, nondistended, well-healed incision.
Genitourinary: no costovertebral angle tenderness, an uncircumcised phallus, and bilaterally descended testicles. A Foley catheter was in place and draining clear yellow urine. Digital rectal exam revealed a prostate size of approximately 70–80 g.

7.2.1.3 Lab Work/Other Studies

– Creatinine was obtained to check the patient's renal function and was at his baseline of 1.2, whereas it had previously been as high as 1.73.
– Urine culture was obtained by sterile straight catheterization and demonstrated >100,000 colonies of *Enterococcus faecalis*. This was treated prior to further urethral instrumentation.
– Cystoscopy was performed in the office and demonstrated a normal urethra without evidence of strictures. The prostatic fossa demonstrated trilobar hypertrophy, causing outlet obstruction. The bladder demonstrated grade 3 trabeculation consistent with high pressure voiding.

7.2.1.4 UDS

See Figs. 7.1 and 7.2.

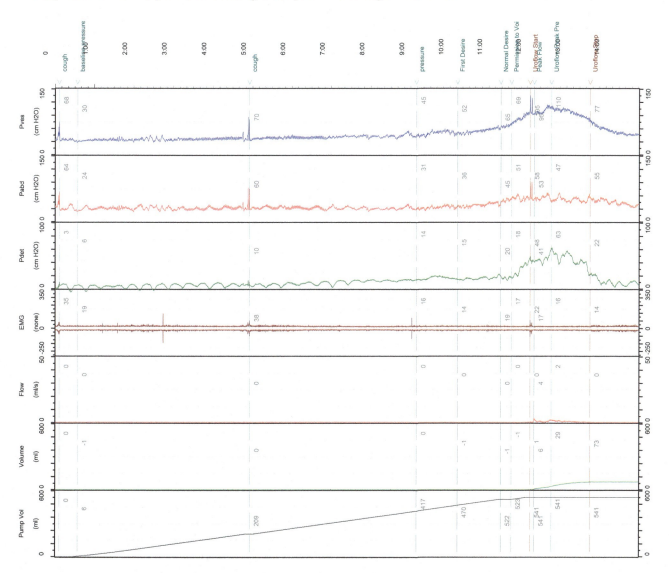

Fig. 7.1 Urodynamics tracing in a patient with Parkinson's disease and urinary retention

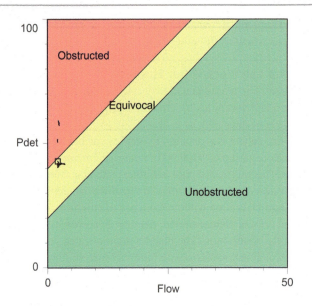

Fig. 7.2 Pressure-flow diagram in a patient with Parkinson's disease and urinary retention

Findings

At the beginning of the urodynamics procedure, uroflowmetry was attempted; however, the patient was unable to void. A Foley catheter was placed for the procedure and 300 mL of clear yellow urine was drained.

Filling Phase

- First desire to void at 470 mL.
- Normal desire at 522 mL.
- Cystometric capacity was 541 mL.
- No DO noted.
- No stress urinary incontinence or urge urinary incontinence.
- Normal compliance.
- Normal EMG activity.

Voiding Phase

- Q_{max} of 3.6 mL/s.
- $P_{det}Q_{max}$ of 62.7 cm H_2O.
- Void a volume of 72 mL.
- PVR was 468 mL.
- EMG activity was synergic.

Urodynamic evaluation in this patient demonstrated decreased bladder sensation with a normal bladder capacity. The uroflow rate was decreased at 3.6 mL/s, and the pattern of flow was plateaued. Detrusor contractility was normal. The patient demonstrated an obstructed bladder outlet and incomplete bladder emptying with a PVR volume of 468 mL. The intravesical voiding pressure was increased at 62.7 cm H_2O.

7.2.1.5 Treatment Options

In this patient who demonstrated decreased bladder sensation, likely secondary to Parkinson's disease, and evidence of BOO, the decision about the best option for treatment must weigh the risks and benefits of surgical options compared to less invasive options. While combined therapy with an alpha-blocker and 5-alpha-reductase inhibitor is a reasonable first option, this patient has failed multiple voiding trials on this regimen after a number of months of treatment. Therefore, an alternative treatment strategy is necessary. CIC would be reasonable in a patient with a limited life expectancy or in a patient unfit to undergo surgical intervention. However, given that this patient has already experienced two urinary tract infections with sepsis requiring hospitalization in a short period of time, surgical intervention is preferable to CIC. In a patient such as this with a moderately large prostate size of approximately 70–80 g, a transurethral resection of the prostate (TURP) is a reasonable option, though a laser vaporization of the prostate could also be considered. Alternative outpatient treatments such as transurethral microwave therapy would be less likely to treat this patient's outlet obstruction adequately.

This patient elected to undergo a TURP. Following the procedure, he was immediately able to void with a PVR volume of approximately 50 mL.

7.2.2 Patient 2

7.2.2.1 History

The patient is a 74-year-old male patient who presented to the outpatient Urology clinic complaining of multiple episodes of urinary retention. This was accompanied by nocturia 4–5 times per night, straining to void, and a weak urinary stream. His primary care provider previously started him on tamsulosin, though he continued to experience episodes of urinary retention with complete inability to void. On initial presentation to the Urology clinic, he was started on finasteride, though after 6 weeks of therapy his PVR volume remained at 75 mL and uroflow demonstrated a reduced Q_{max} of 4 mL/s.

7.2.2.2 Physical Examination

General: no acute distress, appearing his stated age
Psychologic: no signs of depression
Neurologic: no deficits
Cardiovascular: no labored breathing or extremity edema
Abdomen: soft, nontender, and nondistended
Genitourinary: no costovertebral angle tenderness, an uncircumcised phallus, a normal rectal tone, and an approximately 80–90-g prostate on digital rectal exam

7.2.2.3 Lab Work/Other Studies
- Creatinine obtained to check the patient's renal function was 1.7, higher than his previous baseline of 1.
- UA and urine culture were negative.
- A transrectal ultrasound was also performed, demonstrating a 90-g prostate gland.

7.2.2.4 UDS
See Figs. 7.3 and 7.4.

Findings

Filling Phase
- First sensation to void at 87 mL.
- First desire to void at 112 mL.
- Normal desire to void at 158 mL.
- Cystometric capacity was determined to be 355 mL.
- No DO noted.
- No evidence of stress urinary incontinence or urge urinary incontinence.
- Compliance normal.
- EMG activity normal.

Voiding Phase
- Q_{max} was determined to be 4.6 mL/s.
- P_{det} at Q_{max} was 76.3 cm/H$_2$O.
- Voided volume of 175 mL.
- PVR volume was 180 mL.
- EMG activity was synergic.

This urodynamic evaluation in this patient demonstrated a normal filling and storage phase with normal bladder sensation, normal bladder capacity, and no detrusor instability.

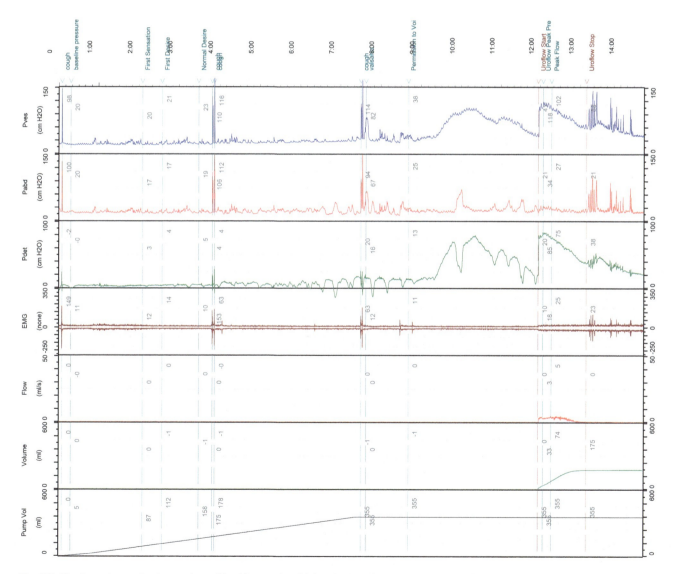

Fig. 7.3 Urodynamics tracing in a patient with a history of multiple episodes of urinary retention and failed dual medical therapy for BPH

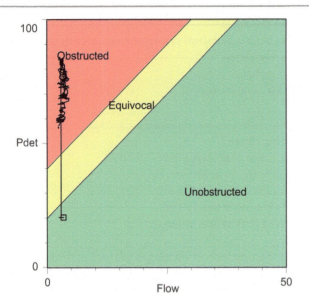

Fig. 7.4 Pressure-flow diagram in a patient with a history of multiple episodes of urinary retention and failed dual medical therapy for BPH

The patient did, however, demonstrate evidence of BOO during the voiding phase of the study. This is evidenced by an increased intravesical voiding pressure and low flow rate. Additionally, the patient demonstrated incomplete bladder emptying. At the end of the procedure, the urodynamics catheter was removed, and the patient was again asked to attempt to void. He was able to void an additional 105 mL at a Q_{max} of 4 mL/s, with a PVR volume of 75 mL.

7.2.2.5 Treatment Options

In patients for whom medical management of presumed BOO secondary to BPH has failed, a thorough assessment of bladder function with UDS and prostate volume should be undertaken. A digital rectal exam may give a crude estimate of prostate volume and should be the initial step in assessing prostate size in these patients. In patients with suspected large volume glands, a transrectal ultrasound may be performed to better quantify the exact volume of the prostate gland and may aid in surgical planning. Additionally, a cystoscopy is a reasonable option to assess bladder and prostate architecture, though it is not necessary. In patients with large volume glands such as this, an open simple prostatectomy has been the standard of care in allowing the greatest amount of adenoma to be removed. Alternatively, as of late, a robotic approach to simple prostatectomy has been described and allows a minimally invasive approach to prostate enucleation [26]. Additionally, some authors have incorporated routine use of holmium and thulium laser fibers to enucleate the prostate adenoma via a transurethral approach. In this case, a holmium laser enucleation of the prostate was undertaken, and a total of 51 g of adenomatous tissue was enucleated. Two years post-procedure, the patient continues to report a significantly improved force of stream and bladder emptying. He has not experienced any additional episodes of urinary retention and continues to have PVR volumes of 0 mL.

7.2.3 Patient 3

7.2.3.1 History

The patient is a 96-year-old male patient with a past medical history remarkable for coronary artery disease and atrial fibrillation, for which he was prescribed aspirin and clopidogrel, who presented to the outpatient Urology clinic complaining of a weak urinary stream, straining to void, and a complete inability to void for the past 12 h. He had previously been diagnosed with BPH and had been prescribed silodosin and dutasteride by his primary care provider. With Valsalva maneuvers, he was able to urinate only a few drops of urine, and a PVR volume measurement demonstrated over 200 mL of residual urine. A Foley catheter was placed at that time and drained 400 mL of clear yellow urine.

Three days after initial catheter placement, the patient returned to the Urology clinic for a trial of void. At this time, however, he was again unable to void, and a Foley catheter was replaced. The decision was made at this time to perform urodynamic testing.

7.2.3.2 Physical Examination

General: no acute distress, appearing his stated age.
Psychologic: no signs of depression.
Neurologic: no deficits.
Cardiovascular: no labored breathing or extremity edema.
Abdomen: soft, nontender, and nondistended.
Genitourinary: revealed a nonpalpable bladder and no costovertebral angle tenderness. Digital rectal exam revealed normal rectal tone and an ~20 g. nontender prostate without evidence of nodularity or induration.

7.2.3.3 Lab Work/Other Studies

– Creatinine of 1.0.
– Urine culture obtained with a Foley catheter in place revealed colonization with *Stenotrophomonas maltophilia*. This was appropriately treated with trimethoprim/sulfamethoxazole prior to urodynamic testing.

7.2.3.4 UDS

See Figs. 7.5 and 7.6.

Findings
Filling Phase
– First desire to void after 135 mL.
– Normal desire to void at 157 mL.
– Cystometric capacity was found to be 177 mL.
– DO noted with UUI event.

7 Bladder Outlet Obstruction: Male Non-neurogenic

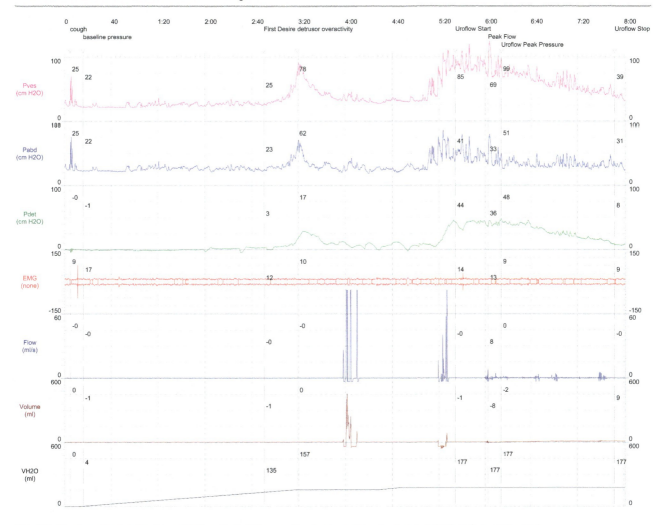

Fig. 7.5 Urodynamics tracing in an elderly patient with a small-volume prostate gland and multiple failed voiding trials

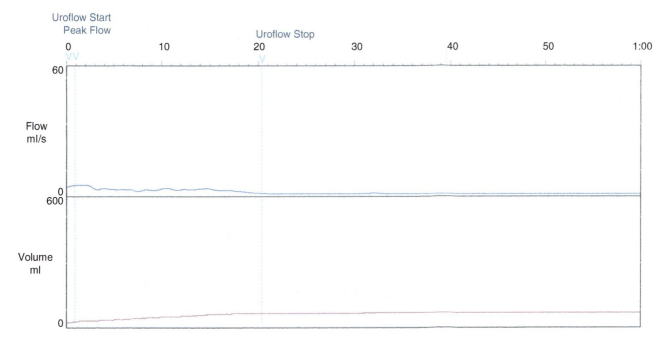

Fig. 7.6 Uroflow tracing in an elderly patient with a small-volume prostate gland and multiple failed voiding trials

- Compliance was normal.
- EMG activity was normal.

Voiding Phase

Of note, the patient was placed in the standing position, as he felt more comfortable voiding this way.

- Qmax 7.8 mL/s.
- $P_{det}Q_{max}$ 48 cm/H$_2$O.
- Voided volume of 30 mL.
- PVR 147 mL.
- EMG activity was synergic.

At this point, the urodynamics catheters were removed, and the patient proceeded to void into the uroflow. This demonstrated a plateaued flow with a maximum flow rate of 4 mL/s and an average flow rate of 2 mL/s. The patient was able to void an additional 43 mL without the urodynamics catheters in place, for a PVR volume of 104 mL.

Urodynamic evaluation in this patient demonstrated normal bladder sensation with decreased bladder capacity. The patient did experience detrusor instability with urge incontinence during the filling phase of the study. The uroflow rate was significantly decreased on the voiding phase of the study, and the uroflow pattern was plateaued. Detrusor contractility was normal, though the patient's intravesical voiding pressure was elevated. He also demonstrated incomplete bladder emptying, with a PVR volume of 104 mL.

7.2.3.5 Treatment Options

Treatment options in elderly patients with BOO secondary to BPH are somewhat limited due to advanced age and comorbidities. Medical management should be attempted primarily as treatment with alpha-blockers and 5-alpha-reductase inhibitors present a relatively low risk and side effect profile. A discussion of the risks and benefits of the various interventions available for BPH must be undertaken with the patient, and the eventual decision on treatment should aim to reduce periprocedural morbidity while affording the patient the greatest opportunity to void spontaneously. Recently developed interventions for the management of BPH, such as the UroLift® System (NeoTract, Inc., Pleasanton, CA, USA), allow a minimally invasive approach that has been shown to improve flow rate and reduce obstructive voiding symptoms in men with BPH. In one systematic review and meta-analysis, International Prostate Symptom Score was found to improve by 7.2–8.7 points, maximum flow rate was found to improve by 3.8–4.0 mL/s, and quality of life improved by 2.2–2.4 [27]. The utility of these interventions should be interpreted with caution; however, given that long-term safety and efficacy data are not available yet.

In this elderly patient with significant comorbidities requiring dual antiplatelet therapy with aspirin and clopidogrel, the decision of treatment modality was based upon minimizing bleeding and providing the greatest relief of outlet obstruction possible. GreenLight™ (American Medical Systems, Minnetonka, MN, USA) photovaporization of the prostate was chosen as it minimizes the risk of bleeding while providing tissue destructive measures to vaporize prostate tissue. Postoperatively, the patient was able to void spontaneously with a PVR volume of 28 mL. He reported significant improvement in his urinary symptoms immediately following the procedure. Two months after the procedure, he experienced an additional episode of urinary retention, and a Foley catheter was required. He did, however, pass a trial of void after 3 days of bladder decompression and has continued to demonstrate low PVR volumes since then.

7.3 Summary

Bladder outlet obstruction in male patients may be the result of numerous different pathologies. Additionally, neurogenic dysfunction of the bladder may mimic BOO and should be considered when the clinical picture suggests it. In young male patients presenting with LUTS suggestive of BOO, strong consideration should be given to urethral strictures secondary to infection or urethral trauma, as well as neurogenic bladder dysfunction. In older male patients who present with obstructive voiding symptoms, consideration should be given to BPH.

Diagnosing an individual patient's pathology should be based primarily on his clinical picture. A history, including past and current urinary complaints, neurologic disorders, pelvic and urethral trauma, previous urologic procedures, family history, and current medications, should be obtained, and a physical exam including a neurologic exam and digital rectal exam is obligatory. Additional diagnostic testing should be tailored to each individual patient's presumed diagnosis.

Urodynamic testing may play a key role in diagnosing and confirming BOO in male patients. Although not required in all cases, numerous clinical scenarios warrant its use. In patients with neurological disorders and in whom BOO is presumed, urodynamic testing allows functional bladder assessment and confirmation of BOO. In patients who have failed treatment for BOO, urodynamic testing allows the urologist to determine whether BOO still exists or if underlying bladder dysfunction is present instead. Therefore, urodynamic testing remains a powerful tool in the urologist's armamentarium when evaluating a patient with presumed BOO.

References

1. Fenter TC, Naslund MJ, Shah MB, Eaddy MT, Black L. The cost of treating the 10 most prevalent diseases in men 50 years of age or older. Am J Manag Care. 2006;12(4 Suppl):S90–8.
2. Berry SJ, Coffey DS, Walsh PC, Ewing LL. The development of human benign prostatic hyperplasia with age. J Urol. 1984;132(3):474–9.
3. Rohr HP, Bartsch G. Human benign prostatic hyperplasia: a stromal disease? New perspectives by quantitative morphology. Urology. 1980;16(6):625–33.
4. Barry MJ, Fowler Jr FJ, O'Leary MP, Bruskewitz RC, Holtgrewe HL, Mebust WK, et al. The American Urological Association symptom index for benign prostatic hyperplasia. The Measurement Committee of the American Urological Association. J Urol. 1992;148(5):1549–57; discussion 64.
5. Jacobsen SJ, Girman CJ, Lieber MM. Natural history of benign prostatic hyperplasia. Urology. 2001;58(6 Suppl 1):5–16; discussion.
6. Fenton AS, Morey AF, Aviles R, Garcia CR. Anterior urethral strictures: etiology and characteristics. Urology. 2005;65(6):1055–8.
7. Lumen N, Hoebeke P, Willemsen P, De Troyer B, Pieters R, Oosterlinck W. Etiology of urethral stricture disease in the 21st century. J Urol. 2009;182(3):983–7.
8. Mundy AR, Andrich DE. Urethral strictures. BJU Int. 2011;107(1):6–26.
9. Meigs JB, Mohr B, Barry MJ, Collins MM, McKinlay JB. Risk factors for clinical benign prostatic hyperplasia in a community-based population of healthy aging men. J Clin Epidemiol. 2001;54(9):935–44.
10. Gacci M, Corona G, Vignozzi L, Salvi M, Serni S, De Nunzio C, et al. Metabolic syndrome and benign prostatic enlargement: a systematic review and meta-analysis. BJU Int. 2015;115(1):24–31.
11. Parsons JK, Carter HB, Partin AW, Windham BG, Metter EJ, Ferrucci L, et al. Metabolic factors associated with benign prostatic hyperplasia. J Clin Endocrinol Metab. 2006;91(7):2562–8.
12. Zhang X, Zeng X, Liu Y, Dong L, Zhao X, Qu X. Impact of metabolic syndrome on benign prostatic hyperplasia in elderly Chinese men. Urol Int. 2014;93(2):214–9.
13. Kang D, Andriole GL, Van De Vooren RC, Crawford D, Chia D, Urban DA, et al. Risk behaviours and benign prostatic hyperplasia. BJU Int. 2004;93(9):1241–5.
14. Platz EA, Kawachi I, Rimm EB, Willett WC, Giovannucci E. Race, ethnicity and benign prostatic hyperplasia in the health professionals follow-up study. J Urol. 2000;163(2):490–5.
15. Abrams P, Chapple C, Khoury S, Roehrborn C, de la Rosette J. Evaluation and treatment of lower urinary tract symptoms in older men. J Urol. 2013;189(1 Suppl):S93–101.
16. McConnell JD, Roehrborn CG, Bautista OM, Andriole Jr GL, Dixon CM, Kusek JW, et al. The long-term effect of doxazosin, finasteride, and combination therapy on the clinical progression of benign prostatic hyperplasia. N Engl J Med. 2003;349(25):2387–98.
17. Kaplan SA, Ikeguchi EF, Santarosa RP, D'Alisera PM, Hendricks J, Te AE, et al. Etiology of voiding dysfunction in men less than 50 years of age. Urology. 1996;47(6):836–9.
18. McVary KT, Roehrborn CG, Avins AL, Barry MJ, Bruskewitz RC, Donnell RF, et al. Update on AUA guideline on the management of benign prostatic hyperplasia. J Urol. 2011;185(5):1793–803.
19. Blaivas JG. Multichannel urodynamic studies in men with benign prostatic hyperplasia. Indications and interpretation. Urol Clin North Am. 1990;17(3):543–52.
20. Nitti VW. Pressure flow urodynamic studies: the gold standard for diagnosing bladder outlet obstruction. Rev Urol. 2005;7 Suppl 6:S14–21.
21. Abrams P, Griffiths D, Hoefner K. The urodynamic assessment of lower urinary tract symptoms. In: Chatelain C, Denis L, Foo K, editors. Benign prostatic hyperplasia. Plymouth: Health Publication; 2001. p. 227–81.
22. Abrams P. Bladder outlet obstruction index, bladder contractility index and bladder voiding efficiency: three simple indices to define bladder voiding function. BJU Int. 1999;84(1):14–5.
23. Abrams PH, Farrar DJ, Turner-Warwick RT, Whiteside CG, Feneley RC. The results of prostatectomy: a symptomatic and urodynamic analysis of 152 patients. J Urol. 1979;121(5):640–2.
24. Oh MM, Choi H, Park MG, Kang SH, Cheon J, Bae JH, et al. Is there a correlation between the presence of idiopathic detrusor overactivity and the degree of bladder outlet obstruction? Urology. 2011;77(1):167–70.
25. Leng WW, McGuire EJ. Obstructive uropathy induced bladder dysfunction can be reversible: bladder compliance measures before and after treatment. J Urol. 2003;169(2):563–6.
26. Sotelo R, Clavijo R, Carmona O, Garcia A, Banda E, Miranda M, et al. Robotic simple prostatectomy. J Urol. 2008;179(2):513–5.
27. Perera M, Roberts MJ, Doi SA, Bolton D. Prostatic urethral lift improves urinary symptoms and flow while preserving sexual function for men with benign prostatic hyperplasia: a systematic review and meta-analysis. Eur Urol. 2015;67(4):704–13.

Bladder Outlet Obstruction: Female Non-neurogenic

William D. Ulmer and Elise J.B. De

8.1 Introduction

Bladder outlet obstruction, well-described in males, is less easily characterized in women. The actual prevalence of obstructed voiding in women is not well known. The EPIC study, consisting of a random sampling of 19,000 adult participants from Canada and four European countries, revealed that 19.5% of the participating women complained of "voiding" lower urinary tract symptoms (i.e., intermittency, slow stream, straining, and terminal dribble) and 59% complained of storage symptoms (i.e., frequency, nocturia, urgency, urge urinary incontinence, stress urinary incontinence, mixed incontinence, and unawares incontinence) [1]. Correlating voiding/storage symptoms with actual obstruction in women has historically been difficult [2], and women with obstruction may additionally present with confounding nonobstructive symptoms. Arriving at a diagnosis of bladder outlet obstruction (BOO) in women requires a detailed medical history and physical exam and a degree of clinical suspicion prior to formal testing.

Urodynamic studies serve as an indispensable diagnostic tool; however, their use and interpretation of the data with respect to female BOO are not well defined. Ultimately, the urodynamic study is used to inform the symptoms, the clinical suspicion, and the surgical and medical plausibility of obstruction. This chapter will present a brief overview of the literature regarding urodynamics for BOO in women and specific case examples regarding interpretation.

8.2 Symptoms of Bladder Outlet Obstruction in Females

Classically, outlet obstruction is characterized by feelings of incomplete emptying, weak stream, intermittency, and hesitancy. These are the result of increased resistance to outflow between the bladder neck and the urethral meatus. Patients may present with voiding symptoms (slow stream, splaying stream, intermittency, hesitancy, straining to void, feeling of incomplete void, or need to immediately re-void) [3]. However, storage symptoms (frequency, nocturia, urge incontinence, urgency) are also common in women with obstruction [1], resulting in a mixed symptom presentation. Obstruction may remain subclinical until the patient presents with an episode of urinary retention (e.g., during the postoperative period for an unrelated surgery), urinary tract infection, or even renal compromise.

8.3 Diagnosis

The work-up for BOO should include an evaluation of postvoid residual, although emptying can be normal. Pertinent history should be obtained regarding prior urological interventions, as the cause of obstruction could be iatrogenic. Providers should screen for neurological disease—diagnosed or undiagnosed—as the bladder function may be impacted and index of suspicion for obstruction is increased. Obstruction is best conceptualized by separating into two categories—anatomic and functional. They are not mutually exclusive and may both be present in the same patient.

8.3.1 Anatomic Obstruction

Anatomic obstruction due to anti-incontinence surgery is the most common cause of BOO in women. It can impact the bladder neck or more distal (mid) urethra. Reported rates of

W.D. Ulmer, M.D. • E.J.B. De, M.D. (✉)
Department of Surgery, Division of Urology, Albany Medical Center, 23 Hackett Blvd, Albany, NY 12208, USA
e-mail: ulmerw@mail.amc.edu; elisede@gmail.com

obstruction in autologous slings vary from 1 to 33% [4], with similar reported rates of intervention (lysis, etc.). Definite obstruction rates are difficult to determine. In the Trial of Mid-Urethral Slings, 46.6% of the women in the transobturator sling group and 42.7% of the women in the retropubic sling group experienced complications of voiding dysfunction, which can be considered a proxy but overestimation of obstruction [5].

Anatomic obstruction in women may be caused by pelvic organ prolapse (particularly stage III or greater) involving the anterior vaginal wall [6]. Descent of the bladder can kink the urethra (if the urethral lateral attachments remain relatively intact) and obstruct urinary outflow. Other less common anatomic causes include benign masses (urethral diverticula or Skene's duct cyst) and malignancies (urothelial or extrinsic mass), stones, ureterocele, urethral stricture, or iatrogenic obstruction due to injectable bulking agents. Urinary retention has been reported in pregnant women due to uterine compression of the urethra [7].

8.3.2 Functional Obstruction

Functional obstruction can result from any impairment of relaxation of the bladder neck or external urethral sphincter. Dysfunctional voiding may result in symptomatic obstruction. Hinman-Allen syndrome is an extreme childhood example in which patients without neurologic abnormalities have failure of relaxation of the external sphincter during voiding, leading to high voiding pressures and overactivity of the detrusor [8]. In adult women, Fowler's syndrome similarly results in failure of external sphincter relaxation. Fowler's syndrome is typically diagnosed in young women in their 20s–30s with findings of elevated post-void residuals (often upward of 1 L without sensation of fullness or discomfort), associated abnormal EMG showing impaired external sphincter relaxation, and discomfort during catheterization (particularly during catheter removal) [9]. Simple high-tone pelvic floor dysfunction including the external urethral sphincter can also present a relative obstruction to the pelvic outlet [10, 11]. Primary bladder neck obstruction (PNBO) is a condition in which the bladder neck fails to open during voiding. This is hypothesized to be due to persistent mesenchyme [12], increased sympathetic tone [13], or functional extension of the striated sphincter to the bladder neck [14]. In one large urodynamic series of women presenting with lower urinary tract symptoms, PNBO was present in 4.6% [15].

Neurogenic causes of obstruction include detrusor-sphincter and bladder neck dyssynergia (multiple sclerosis and spinal cord injury), Parkinson's disease (pseudo-dyssynergia), and other less common neurologic conditions, discussed in a separate chapter. Either the smooth muscle at the bladder neck (bladder neck dyssynergia) or the skeletal muscle at the external sphincter (detrusor-external sphincter dyssynergia) may be affected in neurologic disease. Sirls et al. reported in their series that approximately 25% of their female population with multiple sclerosis were found to have detrusor-external sphincter dyssynergia [16].

8.4 History and Physical Examination

A detailed history is the cornerstone to identifying patients with obstruction. The history should cover chronology, medications, procedures, infections, comorbidities, and injuries. The review of systems regarding back pain, numbness, paresthesias, as well as targeted history regarding urinary tract infection, scoliosis, "bladder lift," and other omitted details can be invaluable. The physical exam should include a post-void residual measurement, pelvic exam to evaluate for organ prolapse, surgical scarring, sling, urethral mass, pelvic floor muscle hypertonicity, evaluation of neurological sensation and reflexes, and urethral hypermobility. There may be a role for cystoscopy, for example, seeking sling obstruction/erosion or primary bladder neck obstruction. Due to the prevalence of both storage and voiding symptoms in women with known obstruction, it is paramount that the evaluating provider maintains an index of suspicion for obstruction during the interview (in particular for patients with a history of genitourinary procedures).

8.5 Role of Urodynamics

Urodynamic testing should not be used as a screening tool. For women with suspected bladder outlet obstruction (with or without mixed voiding symptoms), uroflow and post-void residual testing will provide initial basic data. Urodynamic pressure flow studies with fluoroscopic imaging provide information on bladder neck and external sphincter function, detrusor contraction, Valsalva voiding, and neurological findings such as detrusor-external sphincter dyssynergia. The goal of urodynamic testing for BOO is to demonstrate the classic high bladder pressure and low flow system as well as more subtle findings supporting the clinical suspicion (e.g., dilation of the bladder neck to the level of a midurethral sling on fluoroscopy).

The pressure flow portion of the urodynamic testing can also rule out poor detrusor function as the cause of low flow. Essential to technique is providing secure privacy for the void and enough unhurried time for a true effort. Dim lighting and running water can help, and the examiner should not be in view during the attempts. The examiner should leave the room if needed. A shy voider may be given a diagnosis of atonic bladder if not provided the proper atmosphere for the void. It is not uncommon for a patient with PNBO to be unable to void in public, including during UDS.

The indications for urodynamic studies in the woman with suspected BOO are not well defined. Some authors recommend utilizing urodynamics only once common causes for symptoms are ruled out and initial conservative therapy has failed [4]. For example, preexisting high-tone pelvic floor dysfunction may be exacerbated by sling surgery, leading to frequency and urgency, and a trial of physical therapy may be indicated prior to UDS. Conversely, the patient presenting with obstructive symptoms and elevated post-void volumes immediately after a sling operation for incontinence does not necessarily need urodynamic studies to diagnose outlet obstruction and intervene. In cases where the temporal relationship between obstruction and the surgery are not clear or where the symptoms are more subtle (e.g., pelvic floor dysfunction after a sling), urodynamics may help to elucidate the contributing factors. Urodynamic studies are perhaps most useful in the case of functional obstruction: the history and physical exam are less likely to reveal the cause of obstruction, but properly orchestrated urodynamics may demonstrate the site and sequence of obstruction (e.g., delayed relaxation of the external sphincter in Parkinson's disease). Detrusor-sphincter dyssynergia and dysfunctional voiding may show similar tracings on urodynamics, and both would show obstruction at the level of the external sphincter on fluoroscopy. However, a detailed history and exam (e.g., neurologic disease) and focused testing and trial of intervention (e.g., pelvic floor physical therapy) will distinguish those with presacral neurological lesions. Lastly, urodynamics will show associated pathology, for example, the detrusor overactivity that can develop in the setting of obstruction.

A major issue inherent to the use of urodynamics in the diagnosis of BOO in women is the lack of consensus on a standardized definition. The cutoff values for calculation of obstructive parameters vary [17], and even women with definite obstruction by history and findings (e.g., obstructing sling) may void with detrusor pressures within the "normal" range (such as low pressure voiding) [18]. Several authors have sought to standardize the definition. For example, Blaivas and Groutz developed a bladder outlet obstruction nomogram. Dividing patients into four categories based on the urodynamic maximum detrusor pressure and free uroflow maximum flow rate, they differentiated among the presence, absence, and degree of obstruction [19]. The resulting nomogram distinguishes between moderate (Pdet Max>57 cm H_2O) and severe (Pdet Max>107 cm H_2O) obstruction. However, for lower detrusor pressures (Pdet Max<57 cm H_2O), low flow rates may be seen in the setting of low detrusor pressures in the absence of clinical obstruction. It is the authors' personal experience that most women with obstruction fall in the lower ranges. Chassagne et al. presented standardized cutoff values for obstruction in women [20]. After adjusting for the desired sensitivity and specificity, they calculated the optimal cutoff values for obstructed women to be a PdetQmax between 25 and 30 cm H_2O and a Qmax between 10 and 15 mL/s. When using both, a Qmax of 15 mUs or less and PdetQmax of more than 20 cm H_2O provided a sensitivity of 74.3% and a specificity of 91.1%. Lemack and Zimmern use more strict criteria of Qmax less than 11 mL/s and PdetQmax greater than 21 cm H_2O [21], and Defreitas indicated Qmax<12 mL/s and PdetQmax>25 cm H_2O [17]. Others have illustrated that even some of the best available objective measures of clinical obstruction do not correlate with obstructive symptoms. For example, 47% of Korean women participating in a study reported obstructive symptoms by a standardized pelvic floor distress inventory [22]. Only 34% of those women met obstructive criteria by a value of less than the tenth percentile of peak flow rate by uroflowmetry and 20% by the cutoff values of Qmax less than 12 mL/s and pdet greater than 25 cm H_2O.

Imaging may provide alternative diagnostic assistance. Nitti et al. have demonstrated the usefulness of fluoroscopy in the evaluation for obstruction by employing radiographic obstruction criteria (e.g., the presence of a closed or narrowed bladder neck during voiding in conjunction with elevated post-void residuals and lower than average flow rates). Fluoroscopic imaging can localize the obstruction between the bladder neck and distal urethra in the presence of a sustained detrusor contraction [18]. This can be demonstrated even without application of strict pressure flow criteria and is, in the authors' experience, the most useful approach. Of note, imaging can identify additional pathology such as vesicoureteral reflux.

The varied criteria for obstruction discussed here expose the difficulty in determining outlet obstruction in females. Often, one cannot diagnose clinical obstruction based on urodynamics alone. One must interpret symptoms (voiding and storage symptoms as outlined above), all objective urodynamic parameters, and the available diagnostic tools and algorithms. It is not advisable to use a single parameter to diagnose outlet obstruction, but clinicians can benefit from the use of nomograms such as those discussed in this chapter to support the entire clinical presentation of the patient.

8.6 Case Studies

8.6.1 Patient 1: Primary Bladder Neck Obstruction

8.6.1.1 History

The patient is a 22-year-old female with a long-standing history of voiding problems who failed prior auto-augmentation, interstim, and anticholinergics. She is currently on Ditropan

5 mg IR q am and desmopressin two to three pills at night. She voids spontaneously currently; however, she was on clean intermittent catheterization when she was younger. A recent post-void residual was 425 mL. She has symptoms including small-volume frequent (q 1–2 h) voids with sensation of incomplete void, UUI > SUI, hesitancy, and post-void dribble. She has a history of frequent urinary infections and denies constipation. Sexual function is normal.

8.6.1.2 Physical Examination

Vitals within normal limits. BMI 25.5. Alert and oriented to person, place, and time. Normal mood and affect except for + test anxiety. No acute distress. Heart regular rate and rhythm no murmurs, rubs or gallops. Chest clear bilaterally. Abdomen soft, non-distended, non-tender, and no masses. + Pfannenstiel scar. No costovertebral angle tenderness. No spinal scars. Pelvic: no vaginal atrophy. No uterine, cervical, or vault abnormalities. No appreciable stress incontinence or urethral hypermobility. + High-tone pelvic floor (levator: puborectalis and iliococcygeus) muscles. Nonlocalizing neurological exam, normal anal wink and sphincter tone.

8.6.1.3 Lab Work/Other Studies

Urinalysis—negative for blood, nitrates, leukocyte esterase, and protein.

Urine culture—negative twice prior to referral.

Renal ultrasound—normal right kidney, left upper pole renal scarring—stable over years without hydronephrosis.

PVR 425 mL.

8.6.1.4 UDS

See Figs. 8.1 and 8.2.

Findings

Involuntary contraction was present starting at 113 cm^3. At 138 cm^3 she had an uninhibited contraction (not unusual in the setting of obstruction) to 20 cm H_2O and was able to suppress a leak. At 149 cm^3 she was given permission to void. Detrusor pressure at maximum flow (PdetQmax) was 26, flow (Qmax) 10. By the Blaivas-Groutz nomogram, this puts her in at least the mild obstruction zone. EMG relaxed. Similarly, in Nitti's study, obstructed women were more likely to have a Qmax closer to 9 mL/s. She voided 87 cm^3. Similarly, by the criteria of Chassagne et al. (Qmax < 15 mL/s and PdetQmax > 20 cm H_2O) and Defreitas et al. (Qmax < 12 mL/s and PdetQmax > 25), she is obstructed.

She performed Valsalva at the end which she confirmed was to encourage emptying. PVR was catheterized for 125 mL. Total capacity was therefore 212 mL. In Fig. 8.2, note the hands with rings demonstrating the Crede maneuver

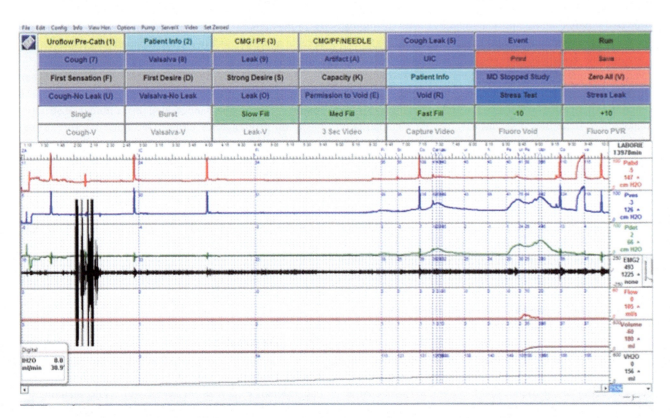

Fig. 8.1 UDS tracing of primary bladder neck obstruction

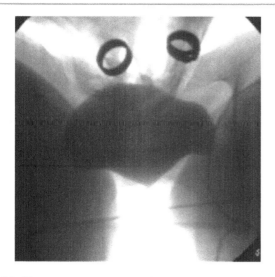

Fig. 8.2 Fluoroscopy demonstrating Crede maneuver to void (rings)

and the closed bladder neck. This image is an excellent example of utility of video (fluoroscopy) urodynamics for demonstrating obstruction during attempted void. Nitti et al. found that video urodynamic obstruction criteria correlate well with standard obstructive criteria [23].

8.6.1.5 Treatment Options

First-line therapies, a trial of alpha blockade and pelvic floor rehabilitation, did not improve emptying. Unilateral transurethral incision of the bladder neck was performed to decrease outflow resistance. The patient maintained anticholinergics for detrusor overactivity. Since stress urinary incontinence is more of a possibility in women after intervention, some women will prefer to self catheterize rather than opt for permanent intervention, and this option should be offered.

8.6.2 Patient 2: Obstructing Sling

8.6.2.1 History

The patient is a 59-year-old woman with a history of pelvic pain who presents for initial evaluation. In 1987, she had a difficult delivery which resulted in "damage in the rectal and bladder areas" with uterine prolapse. She had a hysterectomy in 1991. She experienced voiding symptoms and difficulty with bowel evacuation from 2003 to 2006. She had seen multiple providers over the years for ongoing "voiding issues." In 2007, she had a TVT, vaginal enterocele repair, sacrospinous ligament vault suspension, posterior colporrhaphy with perineorrhaphy, and dermal allograft in the posterior compartment. Later in 2010, she underwent a laparoscopic sacrocolpopexy for vault prolapse and a traction enterocele. Finally, in 2014, she had transanal rectocele repair performed with synthetic material. She presented to our clinic in 2015 due to primarily urinary frequency. She was "worried that [her] bladder is at the wrong angle." The most recent rectocele surgery had aggravated her symptoms. She described LUTS (frequency every 2 h while awake, nocturia × 2–3, weak stream, incomplete emptying, post-void dribbling, intermittency, and posturing/straining to void). She also endorsed urge incontinence and used 1–2 pads per day. She continued to have pelvic pain. The patient underwent a comprehensive evaluation including examination for mesh complications, intervention for high-tone pelvic floor dysfunction, and urodynamic testing.

8.6.2.2 Physical Examination

Vitals within normal limits. BMI 26. Alert and oriented to person, place, and time. Normal mood and affect. No acute distress. Heart regular rate and rhythm no murmurs, rubs, or gallops. Chest clear bilaterally. Abdomen soft, non-distended, non-tender, and no masses. Well-healed surgical scars. No costovertebral angle tenderness. No spinal scars. Pelvic: + vaginal atrophy. Baden-Walker Grade 1 cystocele (POPQ Aa and Ba-2). Some palpable kinking at the level of the TVT. No appreciable stress incontinence or urethral hypermobility. + High-tone pelvic floor (levator: puborectalis and iliococcygeus) muscles with tender trigger points. No mesh erosion. Nonlocalizing neurological exam, normal anal wink and sphincter tone.

8.6.2.3 Lab Work/Other Studies

Urinalysis—negative for blood, nitrates, leukocyte esterase, and protein. Post-void residual volume 100 cm^3 directly post-void.

8.6.2.4 UDS

See Figs. 8.3 and 8.4.

Findings

The patient was found to have normal compliance on the study. Although only 279 cm^3 were instilled, she voided 445 cm^3 and the PVR was 180 cm^3 for a total capacity of 625 cm^3. (Upon questioning she had imbibed a large tea prior to the study.) There was no involuntary contraction. A voluntary contraction was present augmented by some Valsalva voiding. The patient reported (as many do) that she often pushes to augment emptying. Bladder outlet obstruction was judged present, due to pdet > 20 during the void and flow of 10 [Lemack and Zimmern (Qmax < 11 mL/s and PdetQmax > 21 cm H$_2$O), Chassagne et al. (Qmax < 15 mL/s and PdetQmax > 20 cm H$_2$O), and Defreitas et al. (Qmax < 12 mL/s and PdetQmax > 25)] [17, 20, 21], related either to her mild cystocele, the sling, or both. Detrusor-external sphincter dyssynergia was absent as the EUS relaxed during the initiation of the contraction, and the EMG did not rise until she performed Valsalva. There was poor emptying at the end of the study with a PVR of 180 cm^3.

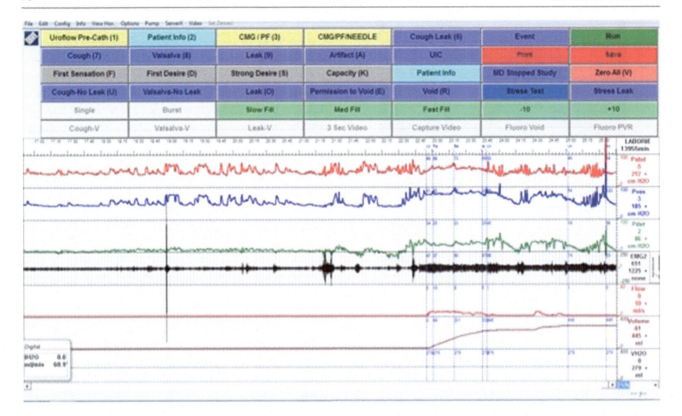

Fig. 8.3 UDS tracing of obstructing sling

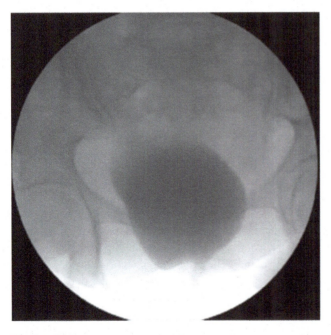

Fig. 8.4 Fluoroscopy demonstrating obstructing sling

Figure 8.4 shows a displaced and kinked bladder neck likely related to a proximal obstructing TVT, with a slight overlying cystocele.

8.6.2.5 Treatment Options

For this complex patient, we performed a trial of pessary prior to sling takedown in order to reassure her that the sling rather than the prolapse was causing the obstruction. She was sent for pelvic floor rehabilitation and treated the urgency with anticholinergics as part of her program given the multiple surgeries and the likelihood of acquired voiding dysfunction related to her pain and obstruction. Additional treatment options would have included intermittent catheterization but given the normal bladder contraction on urodynamics this was down-counseled. Recurrent stress incontinence and worsening of the urge incontinence were advised as risks of urethrolysis.

8.6.3 Patient 3: Obstructing Cystocele

8.6.3.1 History

The patient is a 67-year-old woman who was seen in consultation for pelvic organ prolapse. She was initially referred by her primary physician to a gynecologist who confirmed her diagnosis of cystocele. She stated that she had had trouble with her "bladder dropping." She denied symptoms, but it did bother her to know that the "bulge" was there. She denied LUTS. She did, on further questioning, describe unawares

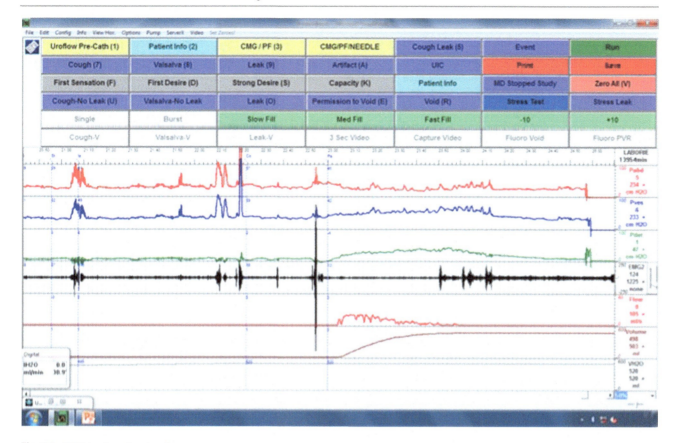

Fig. 8.5 UDS tracing of cystocele

incontinence of two light pads per 24 h, and the odor bothered her.

8.6.3.2 Physical Examination
Vitals within normal limits. BMI 27. Alert and oriented to person, place, and time. Normal mood and affect. No acute distress. Heart regular rate and rhythm no murmurs, rubs, or gallops. Chest clear bilaterally. Abdomen soft, non-distended, non-tender, with no masses. Well-healed lower midline abdominal surgical scars. No costovertebral angle tenderness. No spinal scars. Pelvic: + vaginal atrophy. Baden-Walker Grade 3 cystocele and Grade 1–2 uterine prolapse (POPQ Aa+3, Ba +5, C-3) on supine as well as standing exam. Levator muscles soft, strength three fifths. There was no leakage with cough/Valsalva. Urethral mobility 30°. Normal resistance on catheterization with a post-void residual of 325 mL. Nonlocalizing neurological exam, normal anal wink and sphincter tone.

8.6.3.3 Lab Work/Other Studies
Urinalysis—negative for blood, nitrates, leukocyte esterase, and protein.

Renal ultrasound without hydronephrosis.

Post-void residual urine assessment via catheterization was 325 mL.

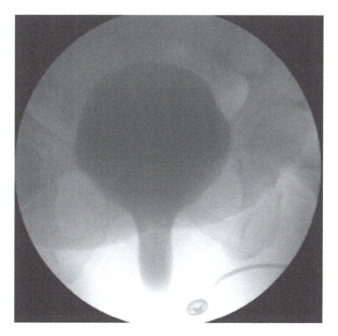

Fig. 8.6 Fluoroscopy demonstrating cystocele

8.6.3.4 UDS
See Figs. 8.5 and 8.6.

Findings

Patient could not void for the free uroflow. The pre-UDS post-void residual was 100 cm^3 by catheterization. On the pressure/flow study, a voluntary contraction was present with detrusor pressure at maximum flow (PdetQmax) of 25 cm H$_2$O while maximum flow (Qmax) was 17 mL/s. Although bladder outlet obstruction was not clearly present by flow, Pdet was 25 cm H$_2$O throughout the void and for 30 s after urination totaling a 60 s contraction. Mild Valsalva was present. These subtle findings, along with fluoroscopic evaluation (Fig. 8.6 showing cystocele by fluoroscopy), were supportive of an obstructing cystocele despite the flow rate being higher than the published algorithms. The cystocele was clearly present 10 cm below the inferior margin of the pubic symphysis on the fluoroscopic images.

8.6.3.5 Treatment Options

The patient was managed initially with a pessary, and we demonstrated improved emptying. She also appreciated dry liners with resolution of the unawares incontinence. There was no new stress incontinence with pessary reduction. She was presented with the option of surgical repair and underwent sacrospinous ligament apical vaginal vault suspension and cystocele repair with plication and cadaveric dermal graft to the arcus tendineus fascia pelvis and sacrospinous ligaments. At follow-up she did very well, with resolution of the bulge as well as the urinary leakage, normal voiding patterns, and the absence of de novo stress urinary incontinence.

8.6.4 Patient 4: Obstructing External Sphincter from Dysfunctional Voiding or Fowler's Syndrome

8.6.4.1 History

The patient is a 42-year-old woman who was seen in consultation for urinary retention, referred by her nephrologist with a creatinine of 3.1 and hydronephrosis on ultrasound. She reported gradual onset of incontinence followed by frank retention, leading to a hospital stay in the United Kingdom in which she was diagnosed with "Fowler's syndrome." She was started on clean intermittent catheterization prior to travel to the United States one month prior to evaluation. She described unawares incontinence, and when the bladder was full she had back pain.

8.6.4.2 Physical Examination

Vitals within normal limits. BMI 30. Alert and oriented to person, place, and time. Normal mood and affect. No acute distress. Heart regular rate and rhythm no murmurs, rubs, or gallops. Chest clear bilaterally. Abdomen protuberant due to adipose tissue. Soft, non-tender, with no masses. No costovertebral angle tenderness. No spinal scars. Pelvic: normal tissues. + Levator muscle hypertonicity. No prolapse. Levator strength unclear as function poorly coordinated—she performs Valsalva rather than contracting. No leakage with cough/Valsalva no urethral mobility. Some resistance on catheterization with a post-void residual of 180 mL. Nonlocalizing neurological exam, normal anal wink and sphincter tone.

8.6.4.3 Lab Work/Other Studies

Urinalysis—negative for blood, nitrates, leukocyte esterase, and protein.

Renal ultrasound + bilateral hydronephrosis, left > right.

Post-void residual urine assessment via catheterization was 180 mL.

8.6.4.4 UDS

See Fig. 8.7a–c.

Findings

Patient could not void for the free uroflow. The pre-UDS post-void residual was 510 cm^3 by catheterization. Compliance was poor at approximately 10, which did not account for the capacitance of the reflux to the kidneys apparent at first imaging at 220 cm^3. This tracing demonstrated artifact due to rectal contractions. Whereas pdet seemed to show bladder contractions, in fact the pves showed a steady slow increase in pressure and it was the artifact from the rectal contractions that affected this appearance. Even after permission to void, there was no change in detrusor pressure beyond the poor compliance. Voiding on the pressure flow study was entirely by Valsalva. She voided 133 cm^3 and post-void residual was 275 cm^3. The surface electrode EMG, using the anal sphincter as a proxy for the external urethral sphincter, was nonrelaxing. Increase in EMG during the actual flow was likely artifact of fluid trickling over the surface electrodes. Bladder outlet obstruction was a more subtle diagnosis in the absence of a distinct detrusor contraction. Rather, in this case, it was the elevated detrusor pressure due to poor compliance (a difference of 40 cm H$_2$O on the pves line versus baseline), the high-tone pelvic floor, and the nonrelaxing sphincter that allowed for the determination.

Additionally, the findings could be consistent with Fowler's syndrome. The patient had a full neurological work-up with no pathology identified. In Fowler's syndrome, increased external urethral sphincter afferent activity due to poor relaxation is thought to inhibit bladder afferent signaling. This can lead to poor bladder sensation and detrusor underactivity. Certainly over time, poor emptying and obstruction can result in poor detrusor compliance. There is some debate regarding whether Fowler's syndrome is distinct from the general category of dysfunctional voiding [24]. Both concepts can be applied to urodynamic interpretation as above.

8.6.4.5 Treatment Options

The patient was retested on high-dose anticholinergics with no improvement. Pelvic floor physical therapy did not impact the

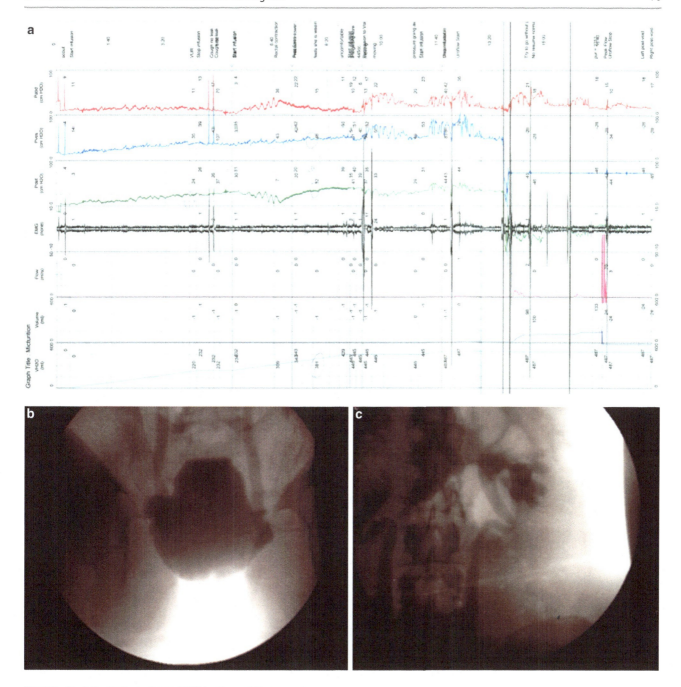

Fig. 8.7 (a–c) Fowler's syndrome UDS tracing and fluoroscopy

voiding patterns. Ileal loop urinary diversion was not an option due to the patient's profession as a performer, and her renal function prohibited augmentation cystoplasty. Due to the markedly impaired compliance and the renal failure, sacral neuromodulation was not entertained as an option. Botulinum chemodenervation of the detrusor was at the time a new treatment. 300U were injected via cystoscope. Repeat urodynamics showed normalization of compliance as well as resolution of the vesicoureteral reflux. The hydronephrosis resolved by ultrasound and the creatinine dropped to 1.8. The incontinence and flank pain resolved. Botox and intermittent catheterization have maintained these results for the past 10 years.

8.7 Additional Points and Related Tracings

1. A poor tracing leads to a poor diagnosis:
   (a) Outside study (Fig. 8.8) failing to establish proper zeros and tracings, failing to appreciate the obstructing cystocele. Provider likely not physically present to observe the exam.
   (b) Repeat study (Fig. 8.9) using proper technique on the same patient showing a clear obstruction.
   (c) The pessary can help minimize the anatomic impact of prolapse. Figure 8.10 shows a tracing on the same patient

after pessary reduction. Although obstruction is still present due either to a too large pessary or an incompletely reduced cystocele, the amplitude of the contraction is less.

2. A good tracing involves zeroing to atmospheric pressure, a cough showing amplitudes of pabd and pves within 70 % of one another and adjusting of the pressure within the rectal balloon to position pdet between 0 and 5 cm H$_2$O. See Fig. 8.11.

3. When a patient has no known neurologic disease and the study looks like neurological disease, investigate. Figure 8.12a, b shows severe obstruction in the setting of detrusor-sphincter dyssynergia in a patient with develop-

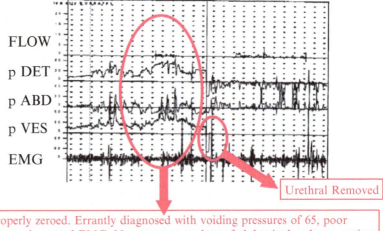

Fig. 8.8 Outside study failing to establish proper zeros and tracings and failing to show obstruction. Female with MUI. Digital evacuation. Large rectocele. Vault prolapse. High cystocele. Prior hysterectomy and cystocele repair

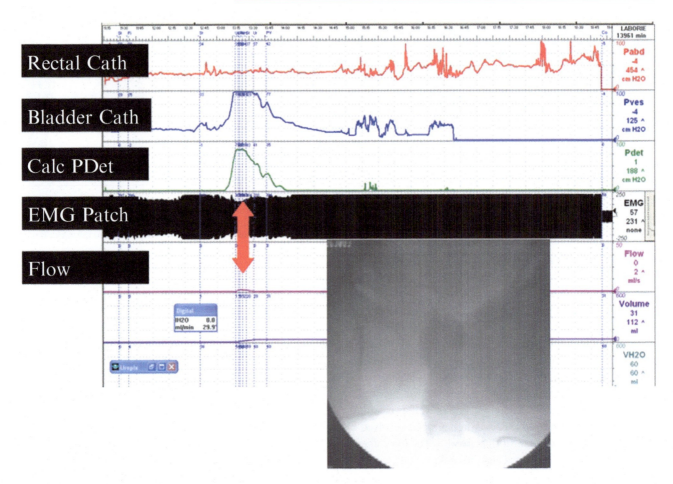

Fig. 8.9 Repeat proper study on patient in Fig. 8.8 showing obstruction. Grade 4 cystocele, vault, and rectocele. BOO

8 Bladder Outlet Obstruction: Female Non-neurogenic

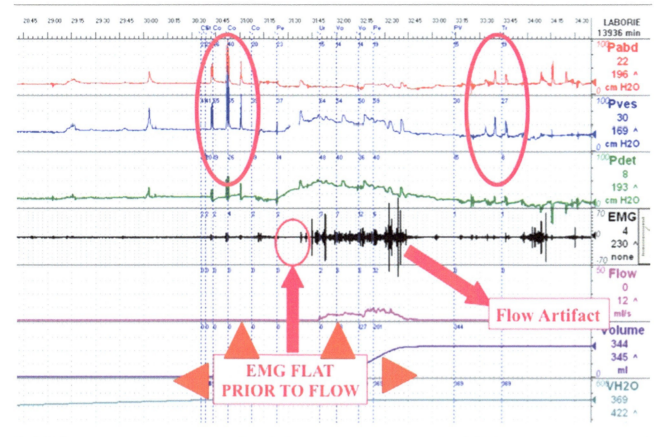

Fig. 8.10 Repeat study with pessary on patient in Fig. 8.8. Pessary can minimize impact of prolapse. EMC flat during contraction prior to void. Slightly high voiding pressure with no abdominal straining. Prolapse repaired

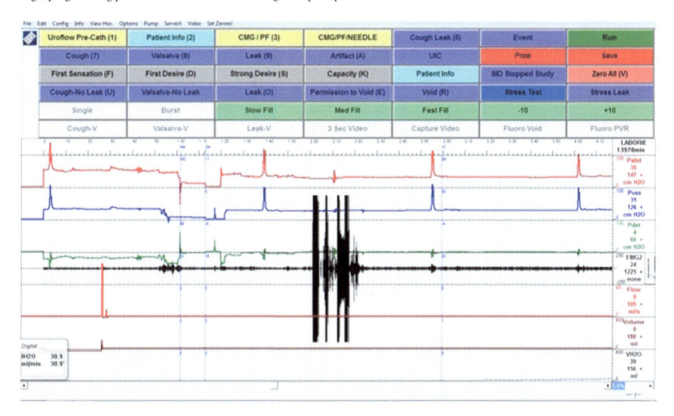

Fig. 8.11 UDS tracing reflective of proper set up for primary bladder neck obstruction, resulting from zeroing to atmospheric pressure, a cough showing amplitudes of pabd and pves within 70 % of one another, and adjusting of the pressure within the rectal balloon to position pdet between 0 and 5 cm H_2O

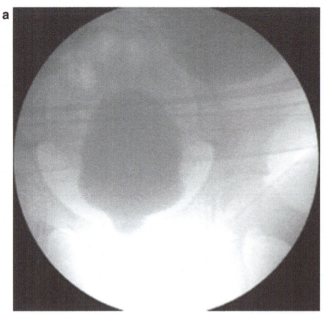
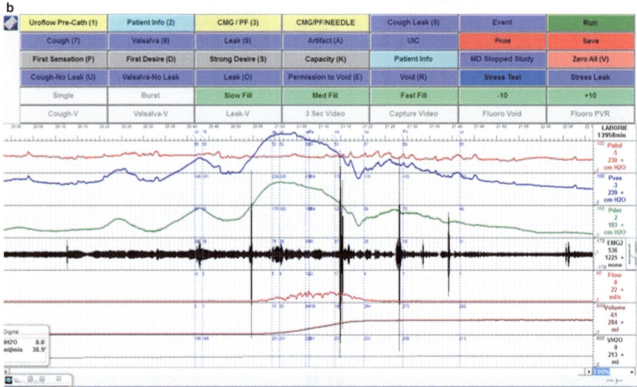

Fig. 8.12 (a, b) Fluoroscopy and UDS tracing showing severe obstruction in the setting of detrusor-sphincter dyssynergia in a patient with developmental delay and previously undiagnosed cervical spine disease

mental delay and previously undiagnosed cervical spine disease.
4. Typically the catheter is too small to obstruct flow, unless there is a stricture rendering the lumen narrow and inflexible. Stricture is rare in women but can be present. See Fig. 8.13.
5. A well-setup study can still be interpretable when the urodynamicist is present to troubleshoot. In Fig. 8.14, the tubing from the pabd transducer and pves transducer was reversed by the technician, but the tracing is still interpretable (obstructed).

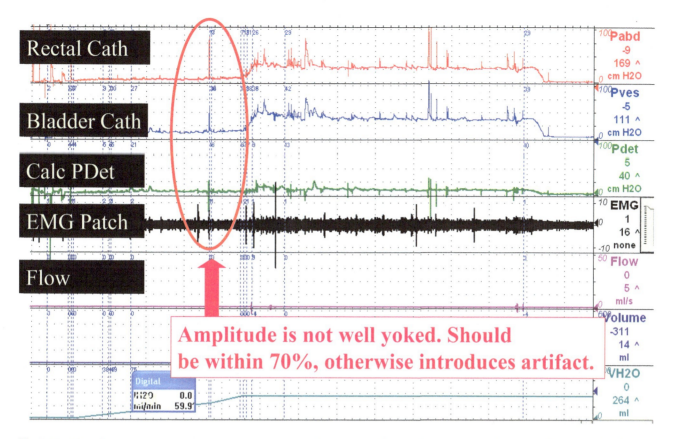

Fig. 8.13 Although a stricture is rare in women, a stricture can render the lumen narrow and inflexible, allowing catheter to obstruct flow. In 8.13, the poor yoking of the catheters gives the pves/pdet the appearance of having a lower amplitude than is actually present. The detrusor contraction is actually more significant, and the patient more obstructed, than appears from the tracing

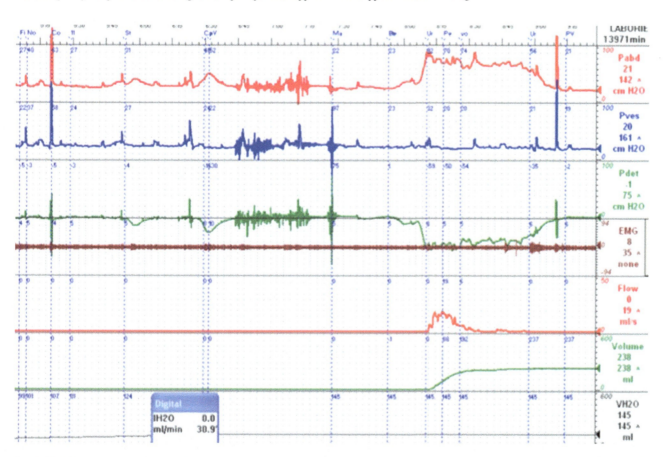

Fig. 8.14 Tubing from the pabd transducer and pves transducer were reversed by the technician in this tracing, but the tracing is still interpretable (obstructed) because the study is well set up

8.8 Summary

The most important components of the urodynamic study are the formulation of the question and setup of the study according to International Continence Society Standards. Without proper zeros and starting pressures or properly reading catheters, it is impossible to make treatment decisions with confidence. In addition, bladder outlet obstruction in women remains a clinical diagnosis supported by evidence from the urodynamic test. The algorithms available for women in the literature are helpful in some cases but cannot be applied to all. The art of the urodynamicist involves synthesizing the relevant clinical information along with the urodynamics tracing to formulate the diagnosis. The required subtleties are facilitated by being physically present for the study.

References

1. Irwin DE, Milsom I, Hunskaar S, et al. Population based survey of urinary incontinence, overactive bladder, and other lower urinary tract symptoms in five countries: results of the EPIC study. Eur Urol. 2006;50(6):1306–14.
2. Lowenstein L, Anderson C, Kenton K, et al. Obstructive voiding symptoms are not predictive of elevated postvoid residual urine volumes. Int Urogynecol J Pelvic Floor Dysfunct. 2008;19(6):801–4.
3. Haylen BT et al. An international urogynecological association (IUGA)/international continence society (ICS) joint report on the terminology for female pelvic floor dysfunction. Neurourol Urodyn. 2010;29(1):4–20.
4. Dmochowski R. Bladder outlet obstruction: etiology and evaluation. Rev Urol. 2005;7 Suppl 6:S3–13.
5. Richter HE et al. Retropubic versus transobturator midurethral slings for stress incontinence. N Engl J Med. 2010;362(22):2066–76.
6. Long CY, Hsu SC, Wu TP, et al. Urodynamic comparison of continent and incontinent women with severe uterovaginal prolapse. J Reprod Med. 2004;49:33–7.
7. Silva PD, Berberich W. Retroverted impacted gravid uterus with acute urinary retention: report of two cases and a review of the literature. Obstet Gynecol. 1986;68:121–3.
8. Nijman R. Role of antimuscarinics in the treatment of nonneurogenic daytime urinary incontinence in children. J Urol. 2004;63(3 Suppl 1):45–50.
9. Hoeritzauer I, Stone J, Fowler C, Elneil-Coker S, Carson A, Panicker J. Fowler's syndrome of urinary retention: a retrospective study of co-morbidity. Neurourol Urodyn. 2016;35(5):601–3.
10. Cheng D. Relationship between anorectal pressure and pelvic floor muscle tension in patients with pelvic floor organ prolapse accompanied by outlet obstruction. Gynecol Obstet Invest. 2011;72(3):174–8.
11. Spettel S, Frawley H, Blais D, De E. Biofeedback treatment for overactive bladder. Curr Bladder Dysfunct Rep. 2012;7:7–13.
12. Leadbetter GW, Leadbetter WF. Diagnosis and treatment of congenital bladder neck obstruction in children. N Engl J Med. 1959;260:633.
13. Crowe R, Noble J, Robson T, et al. An increase in neuropeptide Y but not nitric oxide synthase-immunoreactive nerves in the bladder from male patients with bladder neck dyssynergia. J Urol. 1995;154:1231–6.
14. Yalla SV, Gabilanod FB, Blunt KF, et al. Functional striated sphincter component at the bladder neck: clinical implications. J Urol. 1977;118:408–11.
15. Nitti VW. Primary bladder neck obstruction in men and women. Rev Urol. 2005;7(S8):S12–17.
16. Sirls LT, Zimmern PE, Leach GE. Role of limited evaluation and aggressive medical management in multiple sclerosis: a review of 113 patients. J Urol. 1994;151:946–50.
17. Defreitas GA, Zimmern PE, Lemack GE, et al. Refining diagnosis of anatomic female bladder outlet obstruction: comparison of pressure-flow study parameters in clinically obstructed women with those of normal controls. Urology. 2004;64(4):675–9.
18. Nitti V, Tu LM, Gitlin J. Diagnosing bladder outlet obstruction in women. J Urol. 1999;161(5):1535–40.
19. Blaivas JG, Groutz A. Bladder outlet obstruction nomogram for women with lower urinary tract symptomatology. Neurourol Urodyn. 2000;19:553–64.
20. Chassagne S, Bernier PA, Haab F, et al. Proposed cutoff values to define bladder outlet obstruction in women. Urology. 1998;51:408–11.
21. Lemack GE, Zimmern PE. Pressure flow analysis may aid in identifying women with outflow obstruction. J Urol. 2000;163:1823–8.
22. Jeon S, Yoo E-H. Predictive value of obstructive voiding symptoms and objective bladder emptying tests for urinary retention. J Obstet Gynaecol. 2012;32:770–2.
23. Akikwala T, Fleischman N, Nitti V. Comparison of diagnostic criteria for female bladder outlet obstruction. J Urol. 2006;176:2093–7.
24. Osman NI, Chapple CR. Fowler's syndrome—a cause of unexplained urinary retention in young women? Nat Rev Urol. 2014;11(2):87–98.

Neurogenic Bladder Obstruction

Seth A. Cohen and Shlomo Raz

Abbreviations

ALS	Amyotrophic lateral sclerosis
ALPPs	Abdominal leak point pressures
AD	Autonomic dysreflexia
cm	Centimeters
cc	Cubic centimeter
EMG	Electromyography
CNS	Central nervous system
CVA	Cerebrovascular accident
DSD	Detrusor sphincter dyssynergia
H_2O	Water
MRIs	Magnetic resonance imaging studies
mL	Milliliter
mL/s	Milliliters per second
MS	Multiple sclerosis
MM	Myelomeningocele
PD	Parkinson's disease
pDet max	Maximum detrusor pressure on urodynamics
qMax	Maximum urinary flow on urodynamics
UTIs	Recurrent urinary tract infections
SCI	Spinal cord injury
VUR	Vesicoureteral reflux
VUDS	Videourodynamics

S.A. Cohen, M.D.
Division of Urology and Urologic Oncology,
Department of Surgery, City of Hope,
412 W. Carroll Ave., Suite 200, Glendora, CA 91741, USA
e-mail: cohen.a.seth@gmail.com

S. Raz, M.D. (✉)
Division of Pelvic Medicine and Reconstructive Surgery,
Department of Urology, UCLA, 200 UCLA Medical Plaza,
Suite 140, Los Angeles, CA 90095, USA
e-mail: sraz@mednet.ucla.edu

9.1 Introduction

Neurogenic voiding dysfunction refers to disease pathways impacting the function of the afferent and efferent nerve fibers of the somatic and autonomic nervous systems, which innervate the lower genitourinary tract. The term "obstructive voiding" may in and of itself be misleading, as a neurogenic bladder may be unable to empty, not only because of functional obstruction but because of hypocontractility as well. Thus, perhaps a more comprehensive conceptual framework is to think of this as neurogenic urinary retention. From a urological perspective, when managing these patients, we are not actually treating the disease; we are treating their symptoms. The treatment is based on the ability of the bladder and the urethra to store and empty effectively.

The brain stem is responsible for control of coordinated bladder contraction and pelvic floor relaxation. Cortical and subcortical centers can modulate these sacral reflexes as well [1]. Centers mediating micturition are located within the S2 to S4 sacral area of the spinal cord (including parasympathetic innervation). This part of the spinal cord actually sits at the T12 to L1 vertebral level, which is important to know at times of traumatic injury. Thoracolumbar (sympathetic) output from the T9 to L1 area of the spinal cord also participates in regulation of micturition. As mentioned previously, disturbances of the afferent or efferent innervation pathways can cause neurogenic urinary retention with obstruction being one of these manifestations.

Cortical, subcortical, brain stem, and spinal cord (thoracolumbar or sacral) lesions, in addition to peripheral radiculopathy or neuropathy, can all impact function of the lower genitourinary tract. Neurogenic voiding dysfunction can be complete or incomplete, sensory or motor, central or peripheral, acute or chronic, and reversible or irreversible. It impacts bladder compliance, detrusor activity, smooth sphincter activity, striated sphincter activity, and sensation in varying fashions [2]. Therefore, neurogenic voiding dysfunction can be exhibited as a result of neurologic insults from a wide range of disease processes and trauma: spinal cord injury (SCI), cerebrovascular accident (CVA), multiple sclerosis (MS), Parkinson's disease (PD), myelomeningocele (MM), amyotrophic lateral sclerosis (ALS), diabetes mellitus, acute transverse myelitis, cervical myelopathy, poliomyelitis, tabes dorsalis, pernicious anemia, and sacral root/pelvic plexus surgery (i.e., radical pelvic surgery and spinal surgery) [3].

Of all the described etiologies, MS patients, with detrusor sphincter dyssynergia (DSD), are perhaps some of the most representative of neurogenic obstruction. MS is an autoimmune disease of the central nervous system (CNS) with an extremely variable clinical course. It is described as relapsing-remitting or progressive and is defined by chronic inflammation, gliosis (scarring), demyelination, and neuronal loss [4]. Lesions occur with temporal variability at different locations throughout the CNS. Physiologically, one of the main effects of MS demyelination is to cause discontinuity in saltatory electrical conduction of nerve impulses from one node of Ranvier, the location of concentrated sodium channels, to the next node, resulting in electrical transmission failure [5]. The clinical patterns of MS include the following:

1. Relapsing-remitting (affecting 55–65%, sudden neurologic decline that resolves over 4–8 weeks)
2. Secondary progressive (affecting 25%, develops from relapsing-remitting)
3. Primary-progressive (affecting 10%, most initial symptoms usually motor and continuous)
4. Progressive-relapsing (affecting 5%, aggressive onset with rapid worsening of symptoms) [6]

When evaluating patients with possible neurogenic bladder, including patients with MS, although urodynamic tracings can be completed without a video component, fluoroscopy during these studies offers a rich collection of information, including description of a possible functional obstruction (if it exists and where it is in the tract, i.e., bladder neck, urethra), the state of the bladder (severely trabeculated or smooth), and if there is evidence of high pressures contributing to upper tract deterioration (i.e., vesicoureteral reflux (VUR), dilated ureters). In certain instances, performing a urodynamics study without a video component (or least a post-void residual/bladder scan and a cystogram/upper tract imaging) could be misleading; a decompensated neurogenic bladder with hydroureteronephrosis may have a low filling pressure because the body has already enacted "the pop-off valve" of the upper tract, accommodating for chronically high filling/storage pressures. Without the video component, simply using a cystometrogram tracing to interpret low-pressure filling in a neurogenic bladder may not provide all the important information (the patient may have severe VUR, with associated upper tract dilation). Three case studies will now review various patient presentations, with their associated urodynamic studies.

9.2 Case Studies

9.2.1 Patient 1

9.2.1.1 History

The patient is a 55-year-old gentleman with a history of C5–C6 quadriplegia status post a motor vehicle accident with subsequent cervical fusion (1979), with obstructive sleep apnea, gastroesophageal reflux disease, and neurogenic bladder status post a sphincterotomy (1983), recently with recurrent urinary tract infections (UTIs) and more frequent episodes of autonomic dysreflexia (AD), presenting to clinic for follow-up. He currently empties his bladder through a combination of Valsalva and cutaneous trigger (scratching his thigh with his fingertip or lying supine and tapping his suprapubic area), with urine draining into an external condom catheter he wears at all times.

At times of infection, he develops headaches, chills, diaphoresis, flank pain, and rise in his blood pressure (consistent with his usual AD symptoms). He has been treated for symptomatic UTIs every 2–3 months over the last 18 months, including two hospitalizations for pyelonephritis (presented to the emergency department febrile). He also develops AD at times when his bladder is significantly distended or he is experiencing severe constipation. There is no gross hematuria. His every-other-day bowel regimen includes suppositories, fiber, docusate, and senna. For many years, he has been medically managing his baseline AD symptoms with phenoxybenzamine 10 mg by mouth twice daily. He uses baclofen 20 mg by mouth twice daily for muscle spasm relief. He functions independently and is able to use a motorized wheelchair to get around.

9.2.1.2 Physical Examination

Generally he is in no apparent distress when sitting up in his wheelchair. His upper extremities are contracted, with 3/5 strength and no sensation to light touch (he is not able to hold a pen and squeeze the digits of his hands together). His lower extremities are atrophied. His neck is supple and trachea is midline. Skin is warm and dry. Abdomen is soft, nontender, and nondistended. Genitourinary exam reveals an in-place external condom catheter. The penile skin is intact, with no excoriations. Testes are descended bilaterally, with no palpable masses. Digital rectal exam reveals intact tone, with a 40 g, smooth prostate.

9.2.1.3 Labwork/Other Studies

Post-void residuals as measured by bladder ultrasound were 437 and 397 cc in clinic (additional recent post-void residuals were also documented between 300 and 500 cc). A urine analysis was not checked, secondary to his chronic use of a condom catheter and his lack of symptoms of infection at time of evaluation in clinic. His most recent serum creatinine was 0.4 mg/dL, and estimated glomerular filtration rate (eGFR) was >89 mL/min/1.73 m². A CT of his abdomen and pelvis found no evidence of renal mass, hydronephrosis, or nephrolithiasis. Cystoscopy did not reveal any intravesical abnormalities such as stones, tumors, or diverticula.

9.2.1.4 UDS

See Figs. 9.1, 9.2, and 9.3.

A multichannel videourodynamics (VUDS) was performed in the supine position. The condom catheter was carefully removed without any injury to his penile skin. Initial catheterization revealed a 400 cc residual bladder volume. A rectal catheter was placed for intra-abdominal pressure measurements. A separate 7-French dual-lumen catheter was placed in the bladder. Catheters were zeroed, and filling with Cysto-Conray was begun at 30 cc/min. The filling phase of the study revealed a compliant bladder with low filling pressures. He was able to leak with cough, with abdominal leak point pressures (ALPPs) measured at 60–75 cm H₂O. Initial continuous blood pressure monitoring revealed stable blood pressures ranging from 140/65 to 160/55. As he approached a bladder volume of 600 cc, he started to experience sweats and headache, and another check of his blood pressure revealed it was 180/85. Concerned he was developing AD, the volume infusion was halted.

Fluoroscopic images revealed the bladder neck was open, but his external sphincter did not open. There was no VUR at a volume of 600 mL. He was able to empty another 100 mL with strain. His bladder was then drained of 550 cc. His sweats and headache resolved. His blood pressure returned to 140/65.

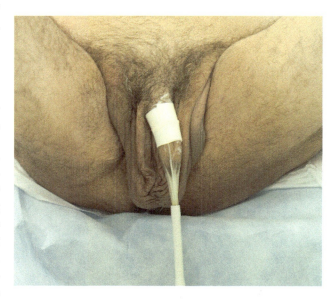

Fig. 9.1 Drainage into an external condom catheter

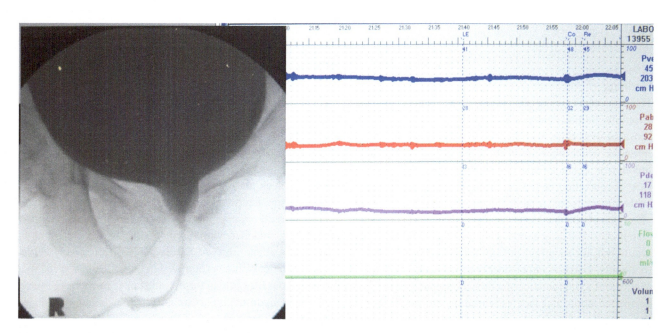

Fig. 9.2 Low pressure filling in a decompensated, hypocontractile bladder

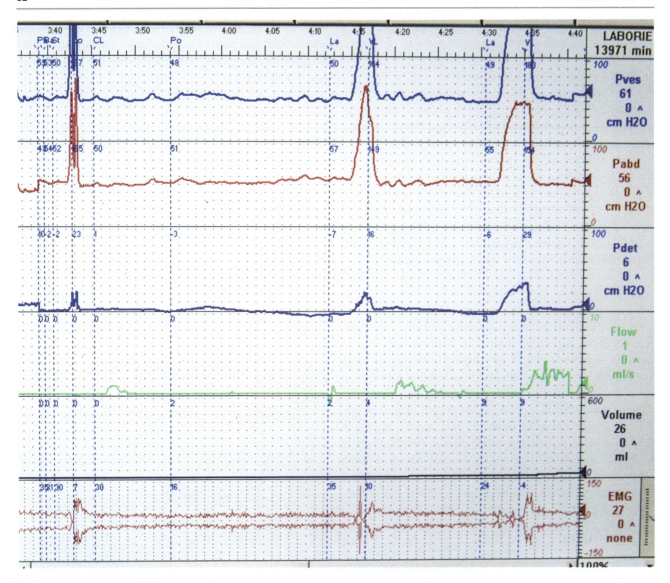

Fig. 9.3 Abdominal leak point pressures

Findings

The patient has normal compliance. Despite previous sphincterotomy, he has evidence of a bladder which has decompensated over time, with hypocontractility, and an external sphincter which does not open. The external sphincter dysfunction is characteristic of a neurological lesion causing lack of relaxation of the pelvic floor. He has no voluntary control over the external sphincter and is not able to completely empty his bladder, with residuals of urine of approximately 300–500 cc at a time. This incomplete emptying puts him at risk for recurrent infection. His AD manifests more frequently, secondary to bladder distension and even more so at times of symptomatic infection. Fortunately, his bladder decompensation and lack of sensation did not impact his upper tract.

9.2.1.5 Treatment Options

He is essentially allowing his bladder to currently empty through overflow incontinence. Management possibilities include the following: commit to intermittent catheterization at least three times a day (but this would require a dedicated caregiver, secondary to his poor dexterity), closure of the bladder neck and creation of an incontinent ileal chimney, another sphincterotomy, or placement of an indwelling catheter (urethral or suprapubic). Considering he is already managing his bladder with urinary leakage into an external condom catheter, he will likely be most effectively served with another sphincterotomy. For now, he has elected to think about his options further; his upper tracts have no evidence of hydronephrosis, renal function is appropriate, he has normal compliance, and there is no VUR. There is not an acute need for immediate action. While awaiting his decision, he will initiate methenamine hippurate 1 g by mouth twice daily, for UTI prophylaxis.

9.2.2 Patient 2

9.2.2.1 History

The patient is a 43-year-old gentleman with a history of MS, neurogenic bladder, incomplete emptying, and persistent urinary urgency, urge incontinence, and frequency, presenting to clinic for follow-up. He manages his bladder with a mix of self-void and self-catheterization, currently voiding every 1–2 h, with occasional urgency urinary incontinence, and catheterizing three times a day, per his report. He has three to four episodes of nocturia per night as well. He had initially tried oxybutynin (both immediate and extended release formulations) without significant improvement in his urinary symptoms. He saw a mild improvement in his urgency and frequency with the combination of tamsulosin 0.4 mg and fesoterodine fumarate 8 mg daily. He takes baclofen 10 mg by mouth twice daily to aid with baseline muscle spasms. He is treated for a UTI every 3–4 months. He denies gross hematuria.

He continues to have some trouble with memory and attention. He denies any changes with vision. He is taking 100 mg of amantadine daily. He continues disease-modifying therapy with glatiramer given subcutaneously three times a week. He continues to take vitamin D 5000 units daily, and his vitamin D level was recently checked by his primary care provider at his annual physical and is reportedly within normal limits. He continues to walk for exercise. Compared to a year ago, there is nothing that he could do then that he is unable to do now.

9.2.2.2 Physical Examination

Generally he is in no apparent distress when sitting up on the examination table. There is full 5/5 strength throughout. Deep tendon reflexes are symmetric and brisk. Sensation to light touch is intact in all dermatomes. Neck is supple. Trachea is midline. Skin is warm and dry. Abdomen is soft, nontender, and nondistended. His lower extremities are atrophied. Genitourinary exam reveals a circumcised phallus and intact glans and meatus. Testes are descended bilaterally, with no palpable masses. Digital rectal exam reveals intact tone, with a 50 g, smooth prostate.

9.2.2.3 Labwork/Other Studies

Post-void residual was not checked, as he catheterizes three times a day to empty his bladder. A urine analysis was not checked, secondary to his intermittent catheterization and his lack of symptoms of infection at time of evaluation in clinic. His most recent serum creatinine was 0.8 mg/dL and eGFR was >89 mL/min/1.73 m^2. Renal ultrasound found no hydronephrosis, obvious masses, or perinephric fluid collections. Cystoscopy did not reveal any intravesical abnormalities such as stones, tumors, or diverticula. MRI imaging of the brain, cervical spine, and thoracic spine documented numerous non-enhancing T2-hyperintense foci scattered throughout the cerebral white matter, posterior fossa, cervical spinal cord, and thoracic spinal cord. No enhancing lesions identified.

9.2.2.4 UDS

See Figs. 9.4, 9.5, and 9.6.

A multichannel VUDS was performed in the upright position. He was initially catheterized for a 70 cc residual (he had voided 20 min prior to the study and self-catheterized 3.5 h before that). A rectal catheter was placed for intra-abdominal pressure measurements. A separate 7-French dual-lumen catheter was placed in the bladder. Catheters were zeroed and filling with Cysto-Conray was begun at 30 cc/min. The filling phase of the study revealed a compliant bladder with low filling pressures. There were multiple short involuntary detrusor contractions associated with urgency multiple times between 174 and 246 cc. He leaked with these contractions at a pDet max of 64 cm H$_2$O, at a volume of 237 mL. At a capacity of 246 cc, he attempted to void and mounted a bladder contraction with a Qmax flow of 6 mL/s, with a pDet max during void of 87 cm H$_2$O, and with a residual of 210 cc. On the fluoroscopic images, there was poor funneling of the bladder neck during attempted void. There was no VUR.

Findings

On the urodynamics, the patient has evidence of a small-capacity bladder, with significant detrusor overactivity associated with urgency urinary incontinence. His bladder neck does not funnel well during voiding, causing inability to empty the bladder. He has normal compliance and no evidence of upper tract damage (i.e., hydronephrosis or vesicoureteral reflux). Considering his underlying MS diagnosis, he may have had chronic obstruction over time from DSD, with subsequent thickening of the bladder wall. A thick, trabeculated bladder wall can contribute to lack of funneling of the bladder neck during attempted void.

9.2.2.5 Treatment Options

His current bladder management of mixed self-void with intermittent catheterization may be yielding a poor quality of life for him. Considering his underlying neurologic dysfunction, any procedure addressing the outlet (i.e., a transurethral incision of his bladder neck or sphincterotomy) would possibly make him even more incontinent. Placement of a suprapubic catheter may create more urinary urgency and urgency incontinence for him. Sacral neuromodulation could be considered, but MS patients often are monitored with MRIs, and

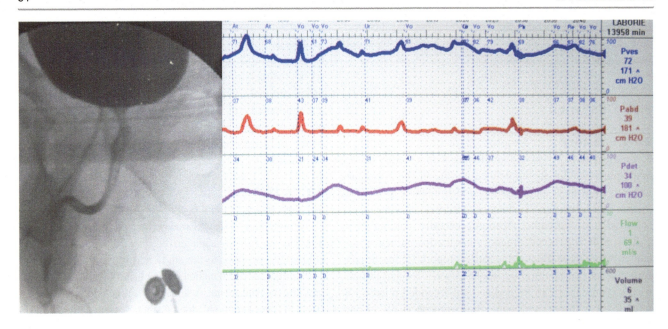

Fig. 9.4 Involuntary detrusor contractions with associated urinary incontinence

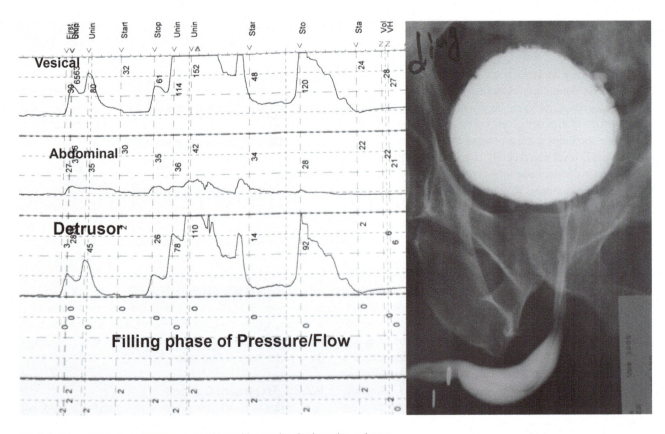

Fig. 9.5 More involuntary detrusor contractions with associated urinary incontinence

the device would prevent him from getting further MRIs. The most reasonable option for him is to try bladder Botox injections to increase the storage capacity of his bladder, with a commitment to increase the frequency of intermittent catheterization to every 3–4 h. If the MS is stable and the Botox fails, augmentation cystoplasty is another reasonable option for him. That would very likely improve his bothersome urgency and frequency. At this time, he has elected to try

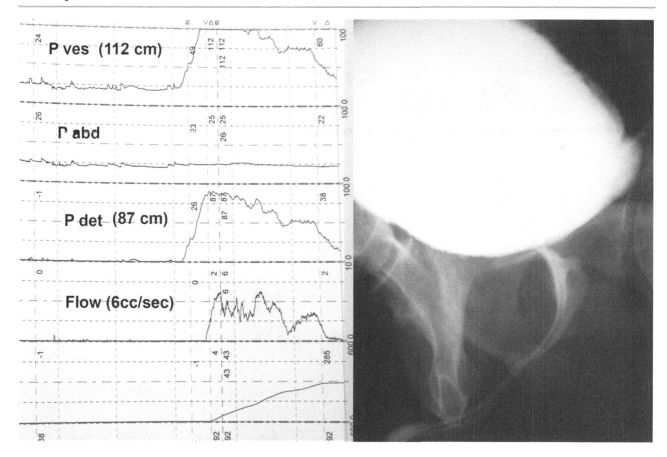

Fig. 9.6 High-pressure, low-flow voiding, with a poorly funneling bladder neck

bladder Botox injections. He will also initiate methenamine hippurate 1 g by mouth twice daily for UTI prophylaxis.

9.2.3 Patient 3

9.2.3.1 History

The patient is a 51-year-old woman with a history of hypothyroidism and a C6–C7 spinal cord injury status post a traumatic fall with subsequent cervical fusion (2013), with neurogenic bladder and urinary incontinence, presenting for evaluation. She is intermittently catheterized twice a day by a caregiver, as she has very poor manual dexterity herself. She cannot catheterize independently. She needs to be transferred to a bed for the catheterization. The availability of her caregiver only allows for the catheterization twice daily. She reports urinary incontinence throughout the day, without sensation of when she is leaking urine. Her urinary incontinence is such that she wears two to three diapers a day. There are no UTIs or gross hematuria. She uses suppositories, docusate, senna, and digital stimulation to aid with chronic constipation. She is very unhappy secondary to her continued dependence on others for her bladder and bowel care. She is able to move about with a motorized wheelchair.

9.2.3.2 Physical Examination

Generally she is in no apparent distress when sitting up in a wheelchair. She has 4/5 strength in her upper extremities, with decreased sensation to light touch in both upper extremities. She is able to hold a pen and squeeze the digits of her hands together. Her lower extremities are atrophied with no sensation and no motor strength. Her neck is supple. Trachea is midline. Skin is warm, dry. Abdomen is soft, nontender, and nondistended. Genitourinary exam reveals normal appearing external female genitalia, with no evidence of significant vaginal prolapse. Digital rectal exam reveals intact tone.

9.2.3.3 Labwork/Other Studies

Post-void residual was not checked, as she catheterizes two times a day to empty her bladder. A urine analysis was not checked, secondary to her intermittent catheterization and her lack of symptoms of infection at the time of evaluation in the clinic. Her most recent serum creatinine was 0.9 mg/dL and estimated glomerular filtration rate (eGFR) was >89 mL/min/1.73 m^2. Renal ultrasound found no hydronephrosis, obvious masses, or perinephric fluid collections. Cystoscopy did not reveal any intravesical abnormalities such as stones, tumors, or diverticula.

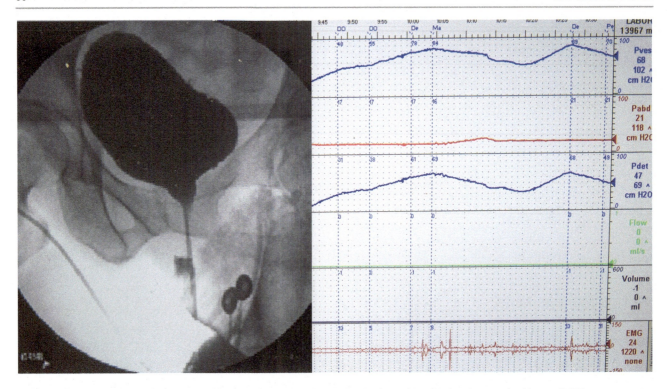

Fig. 9.7 Involuntary detrusor contraction, with subsequent permission to void, in the setting of a closed external sphincter (DSD)

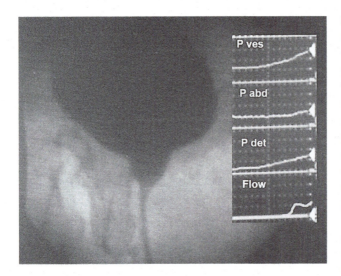

Fig. 9.8 Attempted void, in the setting of DSD

9.2.3.4 UDS

See Figs. 9.7 and 9.8.

A multichannel VUDS was performed in the supine position. She was initially catheterized for a volume of 400 cc. A rectal catheter was placed for intra-abdominal pressure measurements. A separate 7-French dual-lumen catheter was placed in the bladder. Catheters were zeroed, and filling with Cysto-Conray was begun at 30 cc/min. The filling phase of the study revealed a compliant bladder with low filling pressures. An involuntary detrusor contraction at 216 mL, with a pDet max of 61 cm H_2O, was associated with incontinence. During the detrusor contraction, her bladder neck funneled. She was also deemed to have reached capacity at this infusion volume. Fluoroscopic views obtained during the filling phase showed a smooth contoured bladder. There was no cystocele. There was no urethral hypermobility with Valsalva. At rest the bladder neck was closed. With Valsalva, there was no funneling of the bladder neck or incontinence. EMG was performed using surface perineal electrodes. The EMG showed normal activity during filling and increased activity during attempted void; however, during attempted void, she also had lower extremity spasms, and the sensors were wet by this point in the study.

At a capacity of 216 mL, she was already having an involuntary detrusor contraction and was given permission to void; she attempted to void, in the supine position, with the catheter in place at a pressure of 65 cm H_2O with no documented flow. There was no component of abdominal straining. On fluoroscopic images during attempted void, her bladder neck funneled, but her external sphincter appeared to remain closed, consistent with DSD; no urinary stream was visible. Fluoroscopic residual was 300 cc. There was no VUR.

Findings

The patient has a compliant bladder with detrusor overactivity associated with urinary incontinence and DSD. She is unable to empty her bladder. She does not feel the loss of urine with urgency in between intermittent catheterizations, as her neurologic lesion leaves her with no bladder sensation. This is an example of obstruction with severe bladder overactivity.

9.2.3.5 Treatment Options

Catheterizing in a wheelchair can be very challenging for a woman and often requires the patient to transfer to a supine position. She cannot do it without assistance from a caregiver. Although she has DSD, her outlet is still incompetent enough (likely from prior vaginal delivery) that she has urinary incontinence. Management options include a trial of an anticholinergic medication or bladder Botox injections to increase capacity and decrease overactivity, bladder augmentation with creation of a continent catheterizable stoma and closure of the outlet (with either a pubovaginal sling or actual bladder neck closure), an incontinent urinary diversion (a Bricker ileal conduit or an ileal chimney), or placement of a SPT. The option that offers her the greatest opportunity for independence would be the augmentation with creation of a continent catheterizable stoma and closure of the outlet. Her upper extremity dexterity (she can hold a pen and squeeze the digits of her hand together) would be enough for her to catheterize the stoma. This would allow her to avoid diapers and the need for an aide with urethral catheterization. For now, she has elected to think about her options further; her upper tracts have no evidence of hydronephrosis, renal function is appropriate, she has normal compliance, and there is no VUR.

9.3 Summary

When evaluating patients with neurogenic bladder, urodynamics provides important insight, but must be contextualized with additional information, to fully understand the patient's clinical condition. Fluoroscopy images taken during the study (VUDS) allow the provider a window into the upper tracts, to determine if there is VUR or hydronephrosis, and also give the provider the opportunity to assess where a point of obstruction may be (in cases of incomplete emptying). Without imaging the upper tracts, one may evaluate a cystometrogram tracing with low filling pressures and mistakenly presume that the bladder is of reasonable capacity, when in fact there is severe bilateral reflux compensating for a bladder with poor compliance. Without imaging to assess the attempted voiding phase, one may not be able to determine if it is smooth or striated sphincter dyssynergia contributing to obstruction (or perhaps another anatomical finding, such as a urethral stricture). See Figs. 9.9 and 9.10. If not obtaining videofluoroscopic images during the urodynamics study, one should consider at least obtaining a voiding cystourethrogram (VCUG) and upper tract imaging (i.e., renal ultrasound) to contextualize tracing findings.

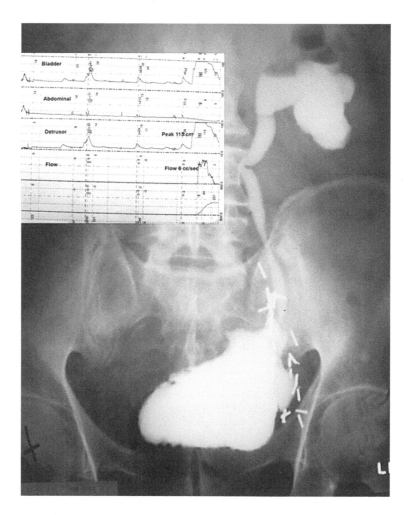

Fig. 9.9 Paraplegic patient with low-pressure filling, but significant left vesicoureteral reflux; during voiding phase, with high pressure, low flow, consistent with obstruction, possibly in the setting of smooth sphincter dyssynergia

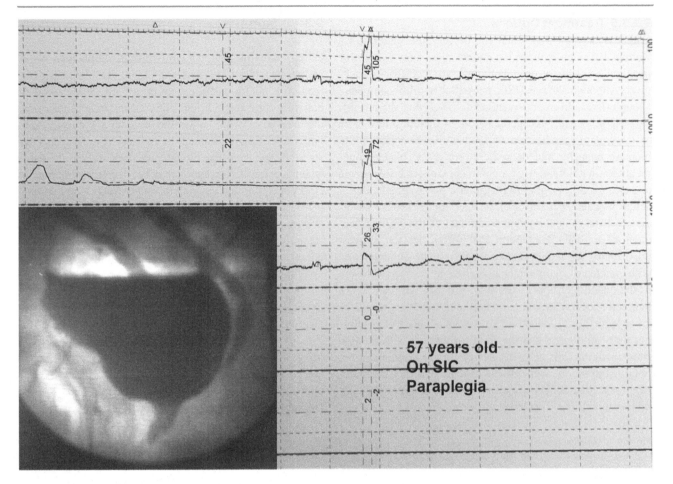

Fig. 9.10 Paraplegic patient, normally performing SIC (self-intermittent catheterization), with low-pressure filling but bilateral significant vesicoureteral reflux

References

1. Waxman SG. The autonomic nervous system. In: Clinical neuroanatomy. 27th ed. New York: The McGraw-Hill Companies; 2013. Chap. 20.
2. Campbell MF, Walsh PC, Wein AJ, Kavoussi LR, Abrams P. In: Kavoussi LR, Wein AJ, et al., editors. Campbell-Walsh urology, vol. 3. 9th ed. Philadelphia: Saunders Elsevier; 2007.
3. Lue TF, Tanagho EA. Neuropathic bladder disorders. In: McAninch JW, Lue TF, editors. Smith & Tanagho's general urology. 18th ed. New York: McGraw-Hill; 2013. Chap. 28.
4. Hauser SL, Goodin DS. Multiple sclerosis and other demyelinating diseases. In: Kasper D, Fauci A, Hauser S, Longo D, Jameson JL, Loscalzo J, editors. Harrison's principles of internal medicine. 19th ed. New York: McGraw-Hill; 2015.
5. Ropper AH, Samuels MA, Klein JP. Multiple sclerosis and other inflammatory demyelinating diseases. In: Adams and Victor's principles of neurology. 10th ed. New York: McGraw-Hill; 2014. Chap. 36.
6. Varacalli K, Shah A, Maitin IB. Multiple sclerosis. In: Maitin IB, Cruz E, editors. Current diagnosis and treatment: physical medicine and rehabilitation. New York: McGraw-Hill; 2015.

Iatrogenic Female Bladder Outlet Obstruction

Sandip Vasavada

10.1 Introduction

Iatrogenic bladder outlet obstruction (BOO) following urinary incontinence surgery is not uncommon. Estimates range from 3 to 43% based on various reports. While the higher numbers may seem excessive and the lower numbers perhaps not representative, there is clearly middle ground from which these cases do arise. The diagnosis of iatrogenic BOO may be elusive. For instance, less often do patients present with classic urinary retention after sling procedures. More often, they have obstructive symptoms such as slow stream, hesitancy, incomplete emptying, or manifestations of this with recurrent urinary tract infections or urgency or frequency. Since there are no agreed-upon parameters of female BOO, we tend to rely on the temporal relationship of symptoms to the incontinence procedures. In other words, if a patient had a sling procedure for stress incontinence and now complains several weeks later of slow stream and straining to void that she did not have prior to the sling, we must consider the sling at fault for creating this scenario [1].

Accordingly, any diagnostic test—be it post-void residual, urodynamics, cystoscopy, or others—would not likely change the time course of events suggesting the sling was to blame. The pelvic surgeon should be readily able to evaluate cases of female BOO in order to optimally manage these patients in the perioperative period. What remains unclear is the longer-term effects of sling surgery that may have created the scenario of female BOO if untreated. Many patients may develop the aforementioned symptoms of irritative and obstructive voiding complaints that now may not respond to simple sling incision. Data are now increasingly available that suggest that these patients are at risk for persistent voiding difficulties if not managed early on after the insult of the surgery [2, 3]. Thus, the consideration at present is to appropriately evaluate suspect female BOO patients early and manage them definitively (early) so as to avoid longer-term complications. That being said, the concern is that of recurrent stress incontinence (often the original presenting complaint) at time of sling surgery, after sling incision. This is clearly a factor both patient and surgeon need to balance prior to embarking upon next step management. The symptoms of bladder outlet obstruction may be anything from irritative voiding symptoms of frequency, urgency, or de novo urge incontinence to frank retention and urinary tract infections. Focused genitourinary examination may demonstrate an otherwise normal exam or even hypersuspension to the urethra or sub-urethral tenderness. One should assess the urinalysis to assure no microhematuria and urine culture if so indicated. Post-void residual urine assessment should be performed in advance of any additional testing as this may be elevated or normal but may guide therapy (if baseline PVR was normal and is now elevated). As previously mentioned, however, a normal or low PVR does not rule out obstruction [4].

10.2 Case Studies

10.2.1 Patient 1

10.2.1.1 History

The patient is a 45-year-old female with no significant past history presenting with complaints of recurrent bladder infections, bothersome urinary urgency and frequency, and new-onset urge incontinence 9 months after an otherwise uncomplicated synthetic retropubic mid-urethral sling for stress incontinence. She has seen by her prior surgeon who diagnosed her with overactive bladder (de novo) and treated her with several anticholinergics and beta-3 agonists without improvement. Her additional complaints include somewhat of a diminished force of stream and nocturia (two times per night) but no stress incontinence. She is now wearing three

S. Vasavada, M.D. (✉)
Department of Urology, Cleveland Clinic,
9500 Euclid Avenue, Q-10-1, Cleveland, OH 44192, USA
e-mail: vasavas@ccf.edu

pads a day and prior to surgery was only wearing one pad unless she was exercising at which point she used up to two pads a day.

10.2.1.2 Physical Examination

The patient has no focal exam findings on general exam. Cardiac exam reveals a slight amount of LE edema, and in psych exam she was alert and oriented to time and place. She had no focal neurologic findings, and her abdomen is otherwise soft and nontender. Her pelvic exam reveals some (<30°) urethral mobility and otherwise no vaginal prolapse. She has no mesh extrusion and no other point tenderness on exam.

10.2.1.3 Laboratory/Other Studies

Urinalysis reveals 0–2 RBC per HPF and no infection.
Post-void residual via bladder scan was 90 mL.

10.2.1.4 UDS

See Fig. 10.1.

Findings

The patient has an otherwise stable cystometrogram (filling phase) and tolerates a normal volume into her bladder (400 cm³). When given permission to void, she has a markedly elevated detrusor pressure (Pdet) of almost 100 cm H_2O with a low flow (5 mL/s). She empties the majority of her bladder with about 100 cm³ post-void residual. At present, there are no completely agreed-upon diagnostic criteria for female BOO. Many use cutoffs of voiding pressure of Pdet > 20 to 25 cm H_2O with a flow of less than 12 mL/s. Others advocate video fluoroscopic views of the outlet to demonstrate proximal urethral dilation with voiding and/or a cutoff or tight area in the mid-urethra corresponding to the location of the sling.

10.2.1.5 Treatment Options

This patient eventually underwent a sling incision. She began, after only a few days, improved flow and less obstructive voiding. Her urgency symptoms improved after a few weeks using some additional behavioral modifications.

10.2.2 Patient 2

10.2.2.1 History

A 66-year-old female presents 6 weeks after a retropubic synthetic sling procedure performed for stress urinary incontinence. Her main complaints are slow stream, straining to void, and hesitancy. She has already had two UTIs since surgery and spends an inordinate amount of time in the toilet trying to void. Her frequency is about every 30 min (up from preoperatively a baseline of every 3 h). Nocturia is new for her at three times a night now. She is increasingly frustrated, and her surgeon has stated to "give it time." An empiric trial of an alpha-blocker was not helpful.

10.2.2.2 Physical Examination

General appearance: No acute distress but frustrated
  Psych: Alert and oriented and frustrated
  Cardiac: RRR and no LE edema
  Neuro exam: No focal deficits

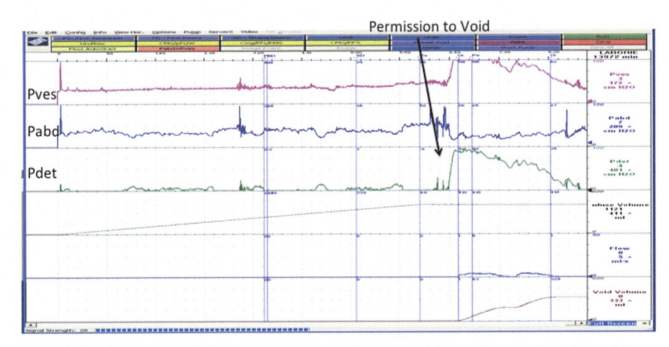

Fig. 10.1 Urodynamics tracing for patient 1

Abdominal exam: Soft, nontender, and nondistended
Genitalia: No prolapse, urethra with mobility to 30°, no mesh exposure, and some point tenderness to urethra

10.2.2.3 Labwork/Other Studies
Urinalysis: 0–3 RBC per HPF, no WBC, and no bacteria
PVR bladder scan: 90 mL

10.2.2.4 UDS
See Fig. 10.2.

Findings
Stable CMG until about 200+ cm³ and then detrusor overactivity; then elevated Pdet with voiding (>50 cm H$_2$O) (voluntary void) and accompanied lower flow rate (12 mL/s)

10.2.2.5 Treatment Options
One can give more time to see if her symptoms resolve, but this is unlikely to get better with time (especially in the case of a synthetic sling). She is clearly obstructed on UDS and will also likely need a sling incision. She should be counseled to recurrent SUI. This may be frustrating for the patient and surgeon, but the long-term sequelae of untreated BOO may be worse with decompensation of the bladder and/or refractory OAB that will not respond to sling incision later down the line.

10.3 Summary

Female bladder outlet obstruction remains a difficult situation to appropriately diagnose. While temporal relationship of new-onset voiding symptoms seems to be the best way to decide upon management now, there may still be a role for urodynamics in less clear cases or those with mixed symptoms etc. Regardless, early therapy may be helpful for the patient in the long run to avoid refractory overactive bladder or persistent voiding dysfunction and its sequelae.

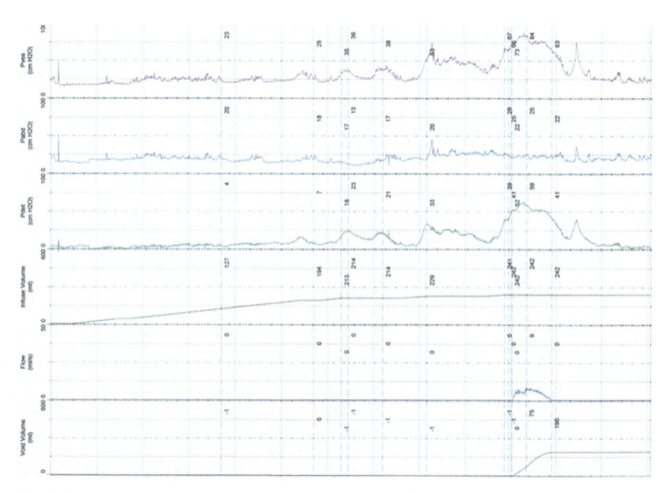

Fig. 10.2 Urodynamics tracing for patient 2

References

1. Abraham N, Vasavada S. Urgency after a sling: review of the management. Curr Urol Rep. 2014;15(4):400.
2. Aponte MM, Shah SR, Hickling D, Brucker BM, Rosenblum N, Nitti VW. Urodynamics for clinically suspected obstruction after anti-incontinence surgery in women. J Urol. 2013;190(2):598–602.
3. Starkman JS, Duffy 3rd JW, Wolter CE, Kaufman MR, Scarpero HM, Dmochowski RR. The evolution of obstruction induced overactive bladder symptoms following urethrolysis for female bladder outlet obstruction. J Urol. 2008;179(3):1018–23.
4. Abraham N, Makovey I, King A, Goldman HB, Vasavada S. The effect of time to release of an obstructing synthetic mid-urethral sling on repeat surgery for stress urinary incontinence. Neurourol Urodyn. 2015. doi:10.1002/nau.22927.

Pelvic Organ Prolapse

Courtenay K. Moore

11.1 Introduction

Pelvic organ prolapse (POP) is a common condition affecting 50 % of middle-aged women [1]. The incidence of POP has been found to increase with age. According to United Nations World Population Aging Data, the number of persons over the age of 60 is expected to double by 2050, totally two billion persons [2]. Given that women over the age of 60 are more likely to seek medical care for pelvic floor disorders, it is estimated that there will be a 45 % increase in the demand for treatment of pelvic floor disorders over the next 30 years [3].

POP is commonly associated with lower urinary tract symptoms (LUTS) including urinary incontinence and incomplete emptying. The effect on POP on LUTS is complex, as it can either alleviate or unmask urinary symptoms. The need for, and utility of, urodynamics in evaluating women with concomitant POP and LUTS is controversial as its impact on postoperative outcomes is highly debated. The questions remain: (1) Can UDS accurately predict which continent women will develop postoperative SUI? And (2) can UDS accurately predict which women POP surgery will alleviate bladder outlet obstruction and improve voiding or reduce PVR?

11.2 POP and SUI

Approximately 50 % of women with POP report preoperative SUI [4]. If left untreated, >60 % of these women will have SUI after POP surgery. Given this high rate of postoperative incontinence, most physicians agree that, in women with concomitant POP and SUI, an anti-incontinence procedure should be performed. However, continent women can also develop postoperative SUI. Upward of 80 % women with occult SUI will develop postoperative SUI [5]. The controversy is which continent women prior to POP surgery should undergo an anti-incontinence procedure, and can UDS accurately predict those women?

In 2006, the landmark colpopexy and urinary reduction efforts (CARE) was published [6]. Three hundred twenty-two stress-continent women with stages 2–4 POP scheduled for abdominal sacrocolpopexy (ASC) underwent UDS with one of five prolapse reduction methods. At the time of ASC, patients were randomized to a Burch colposuspension or no Burch (control) [6].

Preoperatively, only 3.7 % of the patients' demonstrated urodynamic stress incontinence (USI) without prolapse reduction, while 27 % demonstrated USI with POP reduction. At 12 weeks postoperatively, significantly more women in the no-Burch group were found to have postoperative SUI than those in the Burch group (44.1 % vs. 23.8 %). Patients who demonstrated preoperative USI with POP reduction were at a higher risk for postoperative stress incontinence at 3 months, regardless of concomitant colposuspension. However, more patients in the no-Burch group control group were more likely to report bothersome SUI than those in the Burch. In conclusion, the study found that women without stress incontinence who underwent a Burch colposuspension at the time of ASC had significantly reduced postoperative symptoms of stress incontinence. At long-term 5-year follow-up, Burch continued to be protective against SUI [7].

Elser et al. conducted a retrospective review of 441 women also undergoing ASC between 2005 and 2007 [8]. Of the 441 patients, 204 (46.3 %) demonstrated urodynamic stress incontinence with or without POP reduction and underwent an anti-incontinence procedure (Burch or MUS) at the time of ASC. Of these patients, 122 (59.8 %) had UDS SUI and 82 (40.2 %) had occult SUI. Two hundred and thirty-seven (53.7 %) did not demonstrate SUI and underwent ASC alone. At 6-week follow-up, 87.3 % of the women with UDS SUI or occult SUI and 92.8 % of the women with no

C.K. Moore, M.D. (✉)
Glickman Urological Institute, Cleveland Clinic,
9500 Euclid Avenue, Q10, Cleveland, OH 44106, USA
e-mail: mooorec6@ccf.org

preoperative SUI reported no incontinence. Given that UDS diagnosed occult in 40.2 % of those with stress incontinence, the authors conclude that UDS should be performed to determine which patients undergoing ASC require a concomitant anti-incontinence surgery.

Ballert et al. evaluated the role of preoperative UDS in determining the need for a mid-urethral sling (MUS) at the time of transvaginal POP surgery [9]. A total of 105 patients undergoing transvaginal repair for stage 2–4 POP underwent UDS without prolapse reduction. If no SUI was demonstrated, the study was repeated with the POP reduced. Patients underwent a simultaneous MUS if they demonstrated urodynamic SUI or occult SUI. If patients did not demonstrate SUI on UDS with or without POP reduction, a sling was not placed. The risk of intervention for SUI in patients with no clinical, urodynamic, or occult SUI was 8.3 %. In patients who reported a clinical history of SUI but no UDS or occult SUI, the risk for future intervention for SUI is 30 %.

11.3 POP and Bladder Outlet Obstruction

Voiding dysfunction is common in women with POP. Studies have shown that women with advanced POP are more likely to report obstructive voiding symptoms than SUI. Urodynamically, greater than 50 % of women with stage 3–4 POP will demonstrate bladder outlet obstruction (BOO) [10]. Not only do POP stages but also the most dependent portion of the anterior vaginal wall or Ba point correlate with obstructive voiding symptoms [11].

In a study of 60 women with POP stage 1–4, Romanzi et al. found that 75 % of women with stages 3 and 4 POP had evidence of UDS BOO compared to 3 % with stage 1 and 2 POP [10]. While BOO in patients with stage 1 and 2 POP was associated with prior incontinence surgery, it was associated with POP in 94 % of patients with stage 3 and 4 POP. Unlike BOO, detrusor underactivity did not correlate with the degree of POP.

Fletcher et al. retrospectively examined the demographic and urodynamic factors associated with persistent voiding dysfunction after an anterior vaginal wall repair [12]. Preoperatively 29 % of the patients reported difficulty voiding, and of these 87 % had advanced POP. Postoperatively, 74 % of the patients with voiding difficulty reported significant improvement in emptying. Factors associated with improvement in emptying were large PVR and older age, not stage of POP.

While the usefulness of UDS in patients with POP and LUTS is still controversial, in 2012 the American Urological Association/Society of Urodynamics Female Pelvic Medicine and Urogenital Reconstruction issued guidelines regarding the use of urodynamics in the evaluation and management of complex lower urinary tract conditions [13]. Guideline 5 is below:

> In women with high grade POP but without the symptom of SUI, clinicians should perform stress testing with reduction of the prolapse. Multichannel UDS with prolapse reduction may be used to assess for occult stress incontinence and detrusor dysfunction in these women with associated LUTS. (Option; Evidence Strength: Grade C)
>
> A significant proportion of women with high grade POP without SUI symptoms will be found to have occult SUI upon prolapse reduction. If the presence of SUI would change the surgical treatment plan, stress testing with prolapse reduction should be performed to evaluate for occult SUI. This can be done independently or during urodynamic testing. Prolapse can be reduced with a number of tools including a pessary, ring forceps or vaginal pack. The investigator should be aware that the instrument used for POP reduction may also obstruct the urethra, creating a falsely elevated VLPP or preventing the demonstration of SUI.
>
> Multichannel UDS can also assess the presence of detrusor dysfunction in women with high grade POP. UDS with the POP reduced may facilitate evaluation of detrusor function and determine if elevated PVR/urinary retention is due to detrusor underactivity or outlet obstruction or both. Invasive UDS performed both with and without reduction of the POP may help predict postoperative bladder function once the POP has been surgically repaired… [13]

11.4 Case Studies

11.4.1 Patient 1

11.4.1.1 History

The patient is an 87-year-old female s/p TAH/BSO in 1987 followed by anterior and posterior colporrhaphy and perineorrhaphy in 1999 who presents with a 1-year history of a bothersome vaginal bulge. She reports mild urgency but denies UUI and SUI. She occasionally reduces her bulge to "empty better." She cannot remember if she underwent an anti-incontinence procedure at the time of her A&P repair. At some point, she remembers having a mild SUI; however, she currently denies SUI. She denies recurrent UTIs. She is not sexually active and does not desire to be so. She reports diet-controlled hypertension but is otherwise healthy.

11.4.1.2 Physical Examination

General appearance: Normal, no acute distress, and well nourished
Psych: No signs of depression, anxiety, or agitation
Neuro: Gait normal, no UE or LE weakness
Skin/lymph: No rash and lesions
Respiratory effort: Normal, no labored breathing, and lungs CTAB
Cardiovascular: RRR w/no appreciable murmur and no LE edema
External genitalia: +atrophy

Urethral meatus: +caruncle
Urethra: No masses or diverticulum
Urethral angle: <30°, NO SUI with Valsalva or cough with or without POP reduced
POP-Q: Aa=+1, Ba=+2, C=+4, pb=3, gh=4, tvl=7, Ap=+1, Bp=+1, and D=NA

11.4.1.3 Labwork/Other Studies
UA: Negative
PVR: 15 cm^3

11.4.1.4 UDS
See Fig. 11.1a, b.

Findings
For Fig. 11.1a (without vaginal packing):

Filling Phase
CMG: Increased first desire and first sensation
Bladder compliance: Normal
Detrusor overactivity: No
Stress incontinence: No
Maximum cystometric capacity: 250 mL

Voiding Phase
Max voiding detrusor pressure: 21 cm H_2O with void
PdetQmax: 13 cm H_2O, flow at 9 mL/s
Abdominal strain: No
EMG: No DESD or abnormal patterns noted
Impression: Increased sensation and no SUI

For Fig. 11.1b (with vaginal packing):

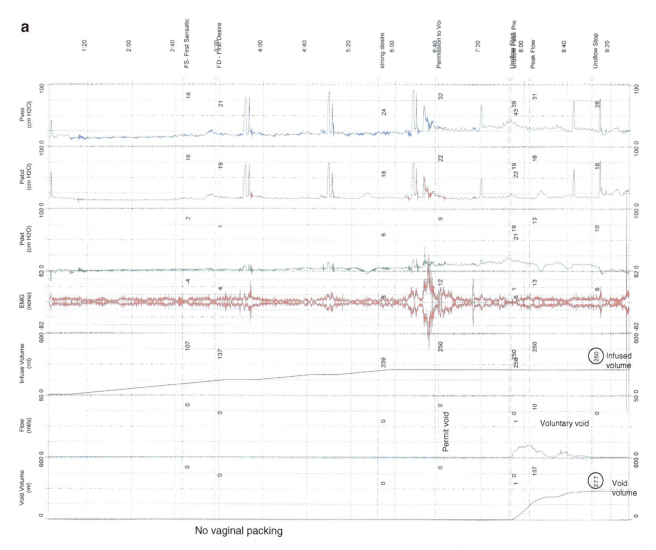

Fig. 11.1 (**a**, **b**) Urodynamics tracings for patient 1; (**a**) without vaginal packing; (**b**) with vaginal packing

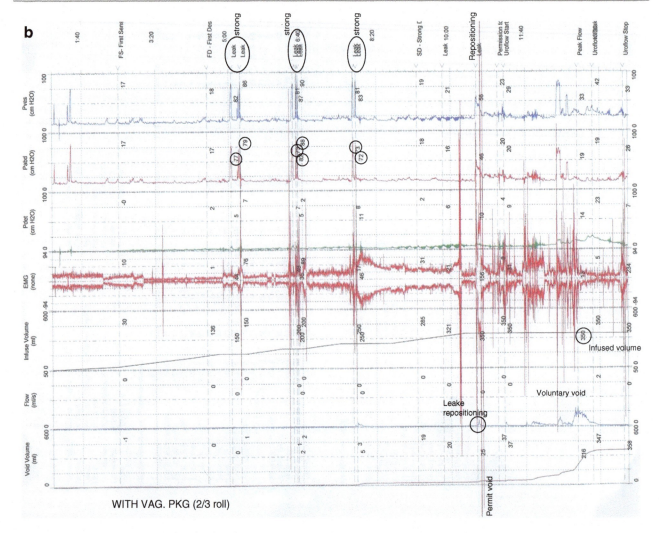

Fig. 11.1 (continued)

Filling Phase
CMG: Early first desire and first sensation
Bladder compliance: Normal
Detrusor overactivity: No
Stress incontinence: Yes
Leaks urine with Valsalva/coughs: Yes
Lowest leak point pressure: 72 cm H$_2$O at 250 mL
Maximum cystometric capacity: 350 mL

Voiding Phase
Max voiding detrusor pressure: 14 cm H$_2$O with void
PdetQmax: 14 cm H$_2$O, flow at 24 mL/s
Abdominal strain: No
EMG: No DESD or abnormal patterns noted
Impression: Early sensation, urodynamic occult SUI reduction of POP

11.4.1.5 Treatment Options

On PE the patient had recurrent stage 3 anterior POP, recurrent stage 2 posterior prolapse, and stage 3 apical prolapse. On UDS the patient demonstrated urodynamic occult SUI. Given that the patient wanted definitive surgical management, sacrospinous ligament fixation, abdominal/robotic sacrocolpopexy, and colpocleisis with a concomitant mid-urethral sling were discussed with the patient. Given that the patient no longer desired to be sexually active, she underwent a colpocleisis and MUS.

11.4.2 Patient 2

11.4.2.1 History

The patient is an 80-year-old female s/p TVH in 2000 and right radical nephrectomy in 2007 for RCC with a 2-year history of a vaginal bulge that has progressively worsened over the last month. Patient reports that since being able to see the bulge her stream is slow and at times she does not feel like she empties to completion. She denies SUI and urgency incontinence but does report an increase in diurnal frequency (daytime frequency × 12 and nocturia × 4) associated with a worsening of the vaginal bulge.

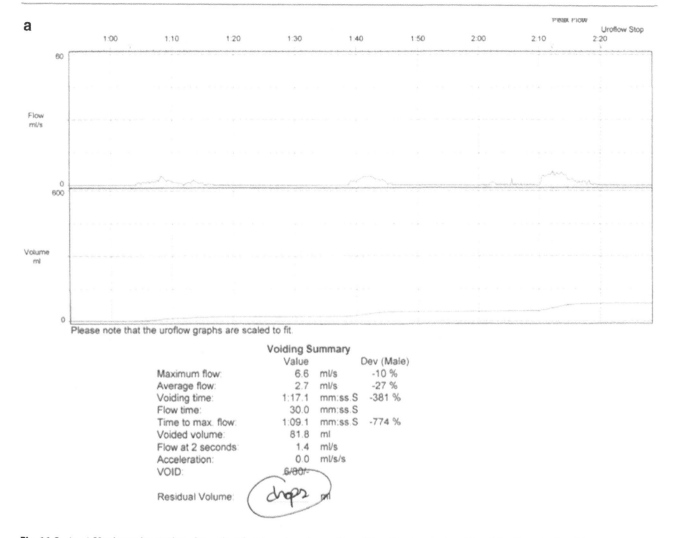

Fig. 11.2 (a–c) Urodynamics tracings for patient 2; (a) noninvasive uroflow; (b) without vaginal packing; (c) with vaginal packing

11.4.2.2 Physical Examination

General appearance: Obese, no acute distress, and well nourished
Psych: No signs of depression, anxiety, or agitation
Neuro: Gait normal, no UE or LE weakness
Skin/lymph: No rash and lesions
Respiratory effort: Normal, no labored breathing, and lungs CTAB
Cardiovascular: RRR w/no appreciable murmur, +LE edema
External genitalia: + atrophy
Urethral meatus: No masses or caruncle
Urethra: No masses or diverticulum
Urethral angle: >30°, NO SUI with Valsalva or cough with or without POP reduced
POP-Q: Aa = +2, Ba = +3, C = 0, gh = 3, pb = 2, tvl = 7 Ap = −2, Bp = −2, and D = N/A

11.4.2.3 Labwork/Other Studies

UA: Negative
PVR: 275 cm^3

11.4.2.4 UDS

See Fig. 11.2a–c.

Findings

For Fig. 11.2a (noninvasive uroflow):

Voided vol: 81.8 mL
Flow time: 30 s
Qmax: 6.6 mL/s
Qavg: 2.7 mL/s
PVR: Drops
Impression: Insufficient volume and intermittent voiding pattern with low flow

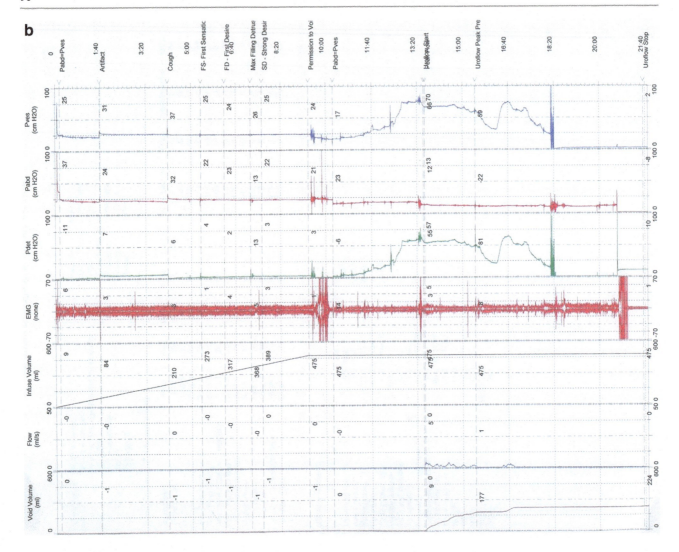

Fig. 11.2 (continued)

For Fig. 11.2b (without vaginal packing):

CMG: Normal first desire and first sensation
Bladder compliance: Normal
Detrusor overactivity: No
Stress incontinence: No
Maximum cystometric capacity: 475 mL
Max voiding detrusor pressure: 57 cm H_2O with void
PdetQmax: 52 cm H_2O, flow at 6 cm^3/s
Abdominal strain: No
EMG: No DESD or abnormal patterns noted
Impression: Elevated voiding pressures and low flow consistent with bladder outlet obstruction

For Fig. 11.2c (with vaginal packing):

CMG: Normal first desire and first sensation
Bladder compliance: Normal
Detrusor overactivity: No
Stress incontinence: No
Maximum cystometric capacity: 400 mL
Max voiding detrusor pressure: 31 cm H_2O with void
PdetQmax: 21 cm H_2O, flow at 9 cm^3/s
Abdominal strain: No
EMG: No DESD or abnormal patterns noted
Impression: Voids to completion with reduced detrusor pressure with reduction of POP

11.4.2.5 Treatment Options

On PE the patient had stage 3 anterior POP, stage 1 posterior prolapse, and stage 2 apical prolapse. On UDS the patient did not have occult SUI and was able to void to completion with reduction of her POP. Given that the patient wanted definitive surgical management, sacrospinous ligament fixation and abdominal/robotic sacrocolpopexy were discussed with the patient. The patient underwent a sacrospinous ligament fixation and an anterior colporrhaphy.

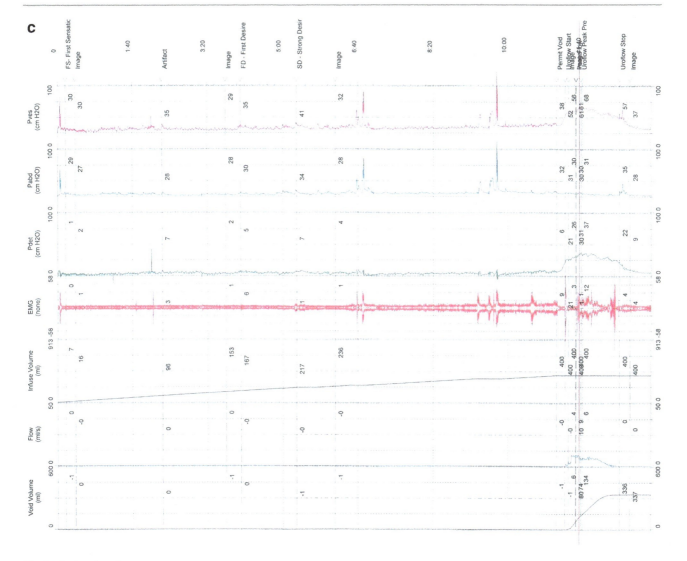

Fig. 11.2 (continued)

11.5 Summary

Women with pelvic organ prolapse have a high rate of concomitant voiding dysfunctions including SUI and obstructive voiding symptoms. Studies suggest that women with POP clinically or urodynamically demonstrated SUI benefit from a concomitant anti-incontinence procedure at the time of prolapse repair. Urodynamics can also help elucidate whether obstructive voiding symptoms and incomplete emptying are related to POP or impaired detrusor contractility. Ultimately, just like any diagnostic test, the use of UDS should be based on whether or not it will help in patient counseling or impact surgical planning.

References

1. Digesu GA, Chaliha C, Salvatore S, et al. The relationship of vaginal prolapse severity to symptoms and quality of life. BJOG. 2005;112:971.
2. United Nations. World Population Aging. 2009; www.un.org/esa/population/publications/WPA2009.
3. Luber KM, Boero S, Choe JY. The demographics of pelvic floor disorders: current observations and future projections. Am J Obstet Gynecol. 2001;184:1496.
4. Lensen EJ, Withagen MI, Kluivers KB, et al. Urinary incontinence after surgery for pelvic organ prolapse. Neurourol Urodyn. 2013;32:455.
5. Svenningsen R, Borstad E, Spydslaug AE, et al. Occult incontinence as predictor for postoperative stress urinary incontinence following pelvic organ prolapse surgery. Int Urogynecol J. 2012;23:843.

6. Brubaker L, Cundiff GW, Fine P, et al. Abdominal sacrocolpopexy with Burch colposuspension to reduce urinary stress incontinence. N Engl J Med. 2006;354:1557.
7. Nygaard I, Brubaker L, Zyczynski HM, et al. Long-term outcomes following abdominal sacrocolpopexy for pelvic organ prolapse. JAMA. 2013;309:2016.
8. Elser DM, Moen MD, Stanford EJ, et al. Abdominal sacrocolpopexy and urinary incontinence: surgical planning based on urodynamics. Am J Obstet Gynecol. 2010;202:375.e1.
9. Ballert KN, Biggs GY, Isenalumhe Jr A, et al. Managing the urethra at transvaginal pelvic organ prolapse repair: a urodynamic approach. J Urol. 2009;181:679.
10. Romanzi LJ, Chaikin DC, Blaivas JG. The effect of genital prolapse on voiding. J Urol. 1999;161:581.
11. de Boer TA, Slieker-ten Hove MC, Burger CW, et al. The prevalence and risk factors of overactive bladder symptoms and its relation to pelvic organ prolapse symptoms in a general female population. Int Urogynecol J. 2011;22:569.
12. Fletcher SG, Haverkorn RM, Yan J, et al. Demographic and urodynamic factors associated with persistent OAB after anterior compartment prolapse repair. Neurourol Urodyn. 2010;29:1414.
13. Collins CW, Winters JC, American Urological Association, et al. AUA/SUFU adult urodynamics guideline: a clinical review. Urol Clin North Am. 2014;41:353.

Augmented Lower Urinary Tract

12

Shilo Rosenberg and David A. Ginsberg

12.1 Introduction

The function of the lower urinary tract is to store and periodically eliminate urine. The lower urinary tract is a low-pressure system and consists of the urinary bladder, bladder neck, and external sphincter. The intact lower urinary tract has important characteristics: normal bladder sensation, capacity, compliance, stability, and voluntary synergistic voiding (pelvic floor relaxation and bladder contraction).

Multiple conditions may disrupt the integrity of the lower urinary tract by changing bladder urodynamic characteristics or pelvic floor synergy. These changes may have a deleterious effect on renal function as a result of increasing bladder pressure and may result in incontinence, incomplete emptying/retention, or other bothersome bladder symptoms such as frequency, urgency, and obstructive voiding symptoms.

The urologist's role in the management of patients with lower urinary tract dysfunction (LUTD) is to correctly assess and treat the underlying pathology or, in some cases, stabilize its effect on the lower urinary tract. The main objectives are to protect renal function, maximize continence, and protect against complications [1].

12.2 Pathophysiology of the Lower Urinary Tract

Various pathologic conditions lead to LUTD. These conditions may be grouped into: neurological, iatrogenic, functional, and inflammatory (Table 12.1). Each etiology may affect the lower urinary tract function differently depending on the site involved or the level of the neurologic insult.

S. Rosenberg, M.D. (✉) • D.A. Ginsberg, M.D.
Department of Urology, Keck School of Medicine at USC,
1441 Eastlake Avenue, Suite 7416, Los Angeles, CA 90033, USA
e-mail: shilo.rosenberg@med.usc.edu; ginsberg@med.usc.edu

The clinical signs of LUTD include incontinence, urgency, frequency, obstructive voiding symptoms, and urinary tract infection. The most important potential adverse outcome related to LUTD is renal failure, which is often the result of decreased bladder compliance and increased detrusor storage pressures. Based on urodynamic studies done in the past on patients with neurogenic bladders secondary to spina bifida, resting bladder pressures greater than 40 cm H_2O place patients at risk of upper tract deterioration [2]. This underscores the importance of periodic urodynamic evaluation and monitoring of patients with neurogenic bladders, since LUTD may change over time. On urodynamic exam, a detrusor leak point pressure (DLPP) above 40 cm H_2O should alert the clinician of a high-risk patient. Treatment is focused on increasing bladder capacity and decreasing storage pressures. This is often achieved by pharmacotherapy (anticholinergics, beta-3 agonists, intravesical botulinum neurotoxin A (BoNT-A) injections) or sacral neurostimulation, with or without clean intermittent catheterization (CIC). However, once less invasive therapies are ineffective, lower urinary tract reconstruction may be required if the patient prefers to manage their bladder with CIC.

12.3 Who to Augment?

The primary goal of augmentation cystoplasty (AC) is a bladder that is a high-capacity, low-pressure reservoir. Potential candidates for bladder augmentation include patients that have failed medical therapy with: DLPP of approximately 40 cm H_2O or higher with signs of upper tract deterioration, incontinence secondary to detrusor overactivity, abnormal compliance leading to urinary incontinence or upper tract damage and severe autonomic dysreflexia secondary to bladder over distension.

Absolute contraindications for bladder augmentation are the inability to perform CIC (by the patient or a caregiver) and the unavailability of bowel [3]. In patients with

Table 12.1 Indications for augmentation cystoplasty

Neurologic		Inflammatory		Functional	Iatrogenic
Acquired	*Congenital*	*Infectious*	*Noninfectious*	Hinman syndrome	Urinary undiversion
Spinal cord injury	Spina bifida	Tuberculosis	Radiation cystitis	Overactive bladder	Vesicovaginal fistula
Multiple sclerosis	Posterior urethral valves	Schistosomiasis	Interstitial cystitis		Loss of bladder tissue
	Extropy/epispadias complex		Chronic cystitis		
	Sacral agenesis				

idiopathic or neurogenic detrusor overactivity, the risk of requiring CIC after augmentation ranges from 39 to 60 % [4, 5]. The decision to augment the bladder in a patient is a multidisciplinary decision with both medical and psychosocial implications. The patient needs to understand and comply with the possibility of a lifelong, strict CIC schedule. Important factors to take into consideration before bladder augmentation are patient independence, habitus, mental illness, reliability, cognitive function, and manual dexterity. On the part of the surgeon, a long-term commitment is required for surveillance and addressing complications if needed.

The choice of segment of gastrointestinal tract used for augmentation depends on the surgeon's experience, renal function, and the presence of factors precluding the use of various segments. In the presence of IBD or irradiated bowel, its use is a contraindication. Oftentimes AC is only one part of an operation where other concomitant procedures are done such as an antegrade enema, catheterizable stoma, and/or a continence procedure for the outlet. This may also affect the decision of what bowel segment to use.

Controversy exists in carrying out AC in patients with renal failure or LUTD as a result of interstitial cystitis (IC)/pelvic pain syndrome (BPS). In patients with end-stage renal disease, debate exists as to the sequence of surgery, that is, should AC be performed before, after, or simultaneously with surgery for renal transplantation. The preference is often to perform the reconstruction prior to renal transplantation.

12.4 How to Augment?

The alimentary tract was first used for AC in 1899 [6]. Initially ACs were carried out for bladder exstrophy or contracted tuberculous bladders. Over the years, the indications for AC have expanded to include all conditions that lead to low-capacity, low-compliance bladders refractory to conservative or minimally invasive therapy. Concepts that evolved over time and made AC a practical solution for patients with threatened upper urinary tracts include:

1. Detubularization of ileal or colonic segments, which increases reservoir capacity and reduces bladder pressure
2. The introduction of CIC which facilitates bladder emptying, especially in neurogenic bladders with detrusor sphincter dyssynergia or acontractile bladders
3. The use of a catheterizable stoma for patients that are unable to perform CIC per their native urethra
4. Procedures to enhance the bladder outlet for patients that have suboptimal sphincteric function, allowing for optimization of continence

Another possibility for AC is the use of the urothelium as autoaugmentation (AA) or ureterocystoplasty. The advantages of augmenting the bladder with urothelial lining are retaining the physiologic barrier and refraining from the use of the alimentary tract and its complications, mainly mucus production, a more elaborated surgery and the risk of bowel complications.

It is difficult to arrive at conclusions regarding the success of these techniques due to a paucity of long-term reports. A study of 47 patients compared patients after AA with AC and a minimal median follow-up of 13 years. There was no difference in continence rate, upper tract status, reservoir compliance, or UTI among groups. However, following surgery, there was a significantly greater increase in bladder volume in patients with AC vs. AA [7]. More recently a study of 25 pediatric patients who had AA and were followed for a median of 6.8 years was published. Four patients had subsequent AC, all but one patient had normal renal function and 18 out of 25 were completely continent. Median bladder capacity at last follow-up was 300 mL and compliance doubled after 1 year to 10 mL/cm H_2O. This article suggested criteria for carrying out AA: 50 % or above estimated bladder capacity for patients' age (or above 200 mL), immediate bladder recycling following surgery, and the surgical technique of hitching the detrusor flaps anteriorly and posteriorly to the rectus muscle and retroperitoneum, respectively, to prevent myotomy closure [8]. Others have not achieved good results and do not recommend this procedure [9, 10].

Since its introduction, intradetrusor BoNT-A injections have gained popularity as a minimally invasive option for the treatment of detrusor overactivity refractory to anticholinergic therapy [11]. Over the last decade, emerging data from clinical trials on patients with neurogenic detrusor overactivity have shown that this modality significantly decreases daily incontinence episodes, improves urodynamic parameters, and leads to clinically meaningful improvements in patient's quality of life. In addition, long-term efficacy has been established with repeated injections, and side effects have been minimal [12, 13]. The increased use of BoNT-A has decreased the need for AC as patients that are refractory to medical therapy now have this option before considering AC [14, 15]. However, in patients with severely decreased bladder compliance/capacity, intravesical BoNT-A injections may not be successful. In one study of 27 patients with NDO treated with BoNT-A, 25 % had persistent urinary incontinence and 20 % ultimately underwent AC. Patients who needed subsequent AC had severely decreased bladder compliance [16].

12.5 Complications of Augmented Reservoirs

Complications of patients following AC are usually divided into early and late.

Early complications are usually related to the surgery itself. Most common early complications cited in the literature include wound infections, vascular events, small bowel obstruction, ventriculoperitoneal shunt infection, and bleeding or persistent reservoir leakage requiring reoperation. CIC is not a complication but an expected consequence of AC [15]. The need for CIC is more frequent in AC due to neurogenic detrusor overactivity (60 %) as compared to patients with idiopathic detrusor overactivity (6 %). The need to perform CIC post-AC appears to increase with time [4].

Long-term complications as a result of AC are not rare and if untreated may lead to morbidity and potential mortality. Metabolic disturbances have been reported as a result of reabsorption of ammonium chloride or secretion of bicarbonate. These disturbances are especially significant in the presence of renal insufficiency/failure. Malignancies in augmented reservoirs have also been described. Most share common features such as a long latency period, a tendency toward adenocarcinomas as the primary histology, and development of the tumor near the enterovesical anastomosis. What is unclear is if this is primarily an issue related to the augment or the native bladder. Recent evidence suggests that congenital dysfunctional bladders are inherently prone to neoplastic transformation and are the primary risk factor for bladder cancer in this patient population [16, 17]. Mucus production may lead to reservoir stone formation and predispose to UTI with a higher incidence in those performing CIC.

Reservoir perforation occurs as a result of overdistension and noncompliance with CIC or may spontaneously occur. Diagnosis is often delayed either due to sensory deficiency in neurogenic patients or "doctors' delay" due to its unfamiliarity among non-urologists [18, 19]. The need for re-intervention following AC is approximately 46 % [20]. Furthermore the need for subsequent open surgery following AC, in patients who need re-intervention, is approximately 50 % [21, 22].

It is important to keep in mind that clinical and radiological signs such as recurrent stone formation, new-onset hydronephrosis, UTI, urinary incontinence, or reservoir perforation may have a common denominator after AC. Poor CIC technique or noncompliance with CIC schedule may give rise to the abovementioned complications. Several studies have shown that the motivation of performing regular CIC dwindles with time [23, 24]. This underscores the importance of regular periodic clinical and radiological evaluation of patients after AC. Occasionally voiding diaries will be needed to assess reservoir functional volume and frequency of bladder evacuation. Urodynamic studies may be necessary to evaluate issues such as urinary incontinence and upper tract changes, which may be secondary to changes (or unresolved problems after the original reconstructive procedure) related to the bladder and/or outlet.

12.6 Urodynamic Studies After Augmentation Cystoplasty

The importance of urodynamic studies prior to AC in patients with LUTD presenting with urgency, frequency, incontinence, or hydronephrosis is clear. The role of urodynamics in neurogenic LUTD, especially in spinal cord injuries, is fundamental. Several studies have shown that managing these patients on the basis of symptoms alone is misleading. Frequently the findings of urodynamic studies do not correlate with clinical symptoms [25–27]. Furthermore, urodynamics has been found to be important in the evaluation of asymptomatic patients with neurogenic LUTD secondary to spinal cord injury. In a study of 80 patients that were followed up for approximately 5½ years with yearly urodynamic studies, it was found that 96 % of patients needed treatment modifications based on these studies. In this cohort the gold standard is videourodynamics (VUD). This modality helps to clarify the consequences of the neurological insult whether it involves the bladder, outlet, or both [28, 29].

The natural history of patients with neurogenic LUTD has changed as a result of the introduction of CIC and the understanding that changes in the lower urinary tract that occur overtime lead to renal failure. Urodynamic studies have a principal role in evaluating these patients [30, 31]. Over the past three decades, in patients with spinal cord injury, the genitourinary tract has shifted from being the major cause of mortality to being the fourth in line [32, 33]. However, even with these innovations, a certain proportion of patients with neurogenic LUTD will fail conservative/minimally invasive treatment and will benefit from lower urinary tract reconstruction.

AC is an outstanding option for patients with a threatened upper urinary tract and incontinence due to refractory DO and poor compliance. Several studies have been published describing the excellent long-term outcomes of patients after

AC. Some studies assessed the long-term durability of the augmented reservoir by urodynamic studies. In a study of 59 patients with heterogeneous causes for neurogenic LUTD followed up for 6.1 years, urodynamic studies were done before and 6 months after operation. Postoperatively mean bladder capacity increased from 220 to 531 mL, and mean pressure at capacity decreased from 48.9 to 15.8 cm H_2O. Complete continence was achieved in 39 patients with persistent incontinence noted in 20 patients (17 mild to moderate, 3 severe). 56 out of 59 patients used CIC. No case of deterioration in renal function was encountered during follow-up, and 53 out of 59 patients were either delighted or pleased with their current state [22].

A study of 26 patients with heterogeneous causes of neurogenic LUTD and a mean follow-up of 8 years had a 96% complete or near-complete continence, and all were managed by CIC. At a mean of 8 years follow-up in 24 out of 26 patients, urodynamic evaluation showed a preoperative to postoperative increase in reservoir volume from a mean of 201 to 615 mL, respectively, and a decrease in maximal reservoir pressure from 81 to 20 cm H_2O. No cases of renal function deterioration were encountered during follow-up [21].

A study of 17 incontinent patients with only spinal cord-related injuries was followed up for a mean of 6.3 years after AC. 15 out of 17 patients (88.5%) were completely continent managed by CIC. Urodynamic evaluation carried out at a mean of 5.4 years showed an increase in mean maximal cystometric capacity from mean preoperative value of 174 mL to a postoperative value of 508 mL and a decrease in mean end filling pressure from preoperative to a postoperative value of 65.5 to 18.3 cm H_2O, respectively. In this cohort during the follow-up period, no case of renal function deterioration occurred [34].

In a recent study of 19 incontinent suprasacral spinal cord injured patients, follow-up was carried out for a minimum of 10.5 years and mean of 14.7 years. All patients were incontinent before surgery and were operated by the same surgeon. Urodynamic data were available preoperatively and postoperatively at 1 year and beyond 10 years of surgery. The maximal cystometric capacity increased from a mean preoperative to 1 and 10 years postoperatively values of 229, 621, and 494 mL, respectively. On the same time scale, a mean maximal detrusor pressure decrease was seen from 81 to 41 and 28 cm H_2O, respectively. Two patients died beyond 10 years of surgery due to unrelated causes. Of the remaining 17 patients, 15 were completely dry. Of the 14 patients that completed a quality of life questionnaire, 13 patients were satisfied and would recommend AC to someone else. No cases of renal function deterioration occurred during follow-up.

The main conclusions of these studies are that the majority of patients will be on CIC following AC, volume increase of the augmented bladder is stable, renal deterioration is prevented over a long period, and continence is greatly improved in the majority of patients. However, an important point to realize is the high rate of re-interventions which underscores the need for long-term surveillance. In these studies the re-intervention rates were up to 35.5–50% [21, 22]. Among the reasons for re-intervention is the need for an additional continence procedure, primarily due to poor urethral sphincteric function that was not identified or addressed at the time of the AC or the need for revision of a catheterizable urinary stoma [35].

What is the yield of performing urodynamics studies in patients after AC? The answer has more to do with expert opinion than clear guidelines. Most authorities would omit regular urodynamic evaluation in continent asymptomatic patients after AC.

In our experience the potential candidates for urodynamic studies after AC would be those that are incontinent following surgery (per the urethra or continent urinary stoma), present with new-onset hydronephrosis, or suffer recurrent reservoir perforation. Incontinence may present immediately after surgery or following several months to years. Candidates for AC are usually evaluated clinically, urodynamically, and possibly endoscopically; however, no one technique is ideal. In a study of 59 neurogenic, incontinent patients who underwent an appropriate pre-AC evaluation, a total of 33% were incontinent following surgery [22].

Assessment of post-AC incontinence should start with thorough history and physical evaluation. When was surgery done? Has there been a neurological deterioration or change? Is incontinence continuous or in drops? Has it worsened over time? Is incontinence at night or diurnal? Incontinence that only occurs during the night is often attributed to changes that may occur during sleep such as a reduction in urethral closing pressure, relaxation of pelvic floor muscles, increase in urine output, and failure of sphincter tone increase in response to contractions in the bowel patch [4].

A voiding diary is extremely helpful to assess functional reservoir volume and frequency of reservoir emptying by CIC. It is not unusual for patients to decrease the interval between catheterizations once they become accustomed to their AC, resulting in excessive volumes when they do perform CIC and subsequent incontinence that is actually a result of elevated bladder volumes and not due to the actual surgical outcome. Following clinical evaluation imaging may be performed. Ultrasound is readily available and provides valuable information of the upper tract. New-onset hydronephrosis may be an indication of increased reservoir pressure.

If a voiding diary rules out poor patient compliance with an appropriate CIC schedule as the cause of the incontinence, then urodynamics should be considered with the focus on bladder filling pressures and the outlet. Several studies have provided evidence of the useful role urodynamics have in assessing patients with incontinence following AC. One study found that 19 out of 323 patients (5.9%) needed re-augmentation due to clinically significant problems originating from the contractile activity of the augmented bladder. These patients presented with a combination of symptoms such as urinary incontinence, recurrent reservoir perforations, and upper tract changes. Urodynamic studies showed high pressure of above 40 cm H_2O at less than 200 mL with rhythmic contractions in 12 patients, small-capacity reservoir in three patients, and a poorly compliant bladder in one patient. In 95 % of patients, complete continence was achieved by re-augmentation [36].

Stress urinary incontinence (SUI) following AC maybe caused by an inadequate augment; however, more common is the failure to recognize an incompetent outlet during preoperative evaluation. In one study 11 % of patients suffered from SUI following AC [34]. Potential reasons for not diagnosing patients with an incompetent outlet include technically difficult to evaluate a low-capacity, low-compliance bladder and overlooking the poor sphincteric function, assuming deturor overactivity or poor compliance is the sole cause of a patient's leakage and not also evaluating the outlet during a urodynamic study, and inability to adequately evaluate the outlet if undiversion is planned for a patient who, for example, had their urine diverted to an ileal conduit following pelvic trauma, with or without spinal cord injury. Most incontinent patients with neurogenic bladders will gain continence by AC alone [4, 37]. In the minority who suffer from urinary incontinence following AC, UDS have been found to be reliable in diagnosing bladder outlet incompetence if it is present. Several studies have been published that utilize various urodynamic parameters such as bladder outlet morphology at 20 cm H_2O, static leak point pressure or Valsalva leak point pressure. One study evaluated 26 patients with neurogenic bladders who failed conservative therapy and underwent subsequent AC, 19 of whom were incontinent before AC. Following surgery four patients remained incontinent; the pre-op VUD findings in these four incontinent patients included an open bladder neck at a pressure of 20 cm H_2O [38].

Others have found VUD not useful in the standard evaluation of patients after AC. One study investigated 50 patients with neuropathic bladders and 50 with unstable bladders before and after AC with no other additional procedures. VUD studies were performed before and after AC. The results showed that the inherent qualities of the bowel and especially the neurogenic bowel make urodynamic evaluation less relevant in patients after augmentation. Bowel contracts regularly and involuntarily, and these traits increase at higher wall tension. So although results of urodynamic studies may show overactivity and decreased compliance, it has little correlation with clinical symptoms. The conclusions of this study were that ultrasound is as valuable as urodynamics and less invasive to assess the upper and lower urinary tract post-AC, the bowel-augmented bladder protects the upper tract by increasing capacity, and if one avoids reaching the upper extreme of capacity, the decreased compliance and increased contractility are prevented [39]. What is not clear is how the patient or the physician knows what is the "upper extremity" of the capacity. Clearly most patients do fine with AC, and if they remain dry and have stable upper urinary tracts, further urodynamic evaluation post-AC is often not helpful. However, urodynamics is certainly a useful tool to evaluate patients' post-AC who have appropriate indications.

12.7 Case Studies

12.7.1 Patient 1

A 24-year-old male had augmentation cystoplasty and some unknown type of bladder neck reconstruction as a child. He has UI despite CIC q4 h. No upper tract changes were seen. There was no improvement with solifenacin. Urodynamic studies were done (Fig. 12.1). The study shows loss of compliance with filling and a competent outlet. His lower urinary tract was re-augmented with resolution of his incontinence.

12.7.2 Patient 2

A 45-year-old male had a history of T12 spinal cord injury. He complained of urinary incontinence despite maximal medical therapy and ultimately underwent AC. Following surgery urinary incontinence persisted. Videourodynamic studies done show a high-volume, low-pressure system. Stress urinary incontinence is evident as denoted by leak with Valsalva (Fig. 12.2). The fluoroscopic image (Fig. 12.3) displays urinary leakage during Valsalva at a volume of 150 and 375 mL. In this case this patient's outlet incompetence was not diagnosed preoperatively. Treatment of his stress incontinence was done with placement of an artificial urinary sphincter.

12.8 Summary

In summary, being nonphysiologic, AC with bowel is a compromise. Although it fulfills its primary indication of renal protection, the consequences of this procedure also puts a patient in need of lifelong medical surveillance with a realistic chance of subsequent minimally invasive or surgical interventions. Still most patients accept this trade-off. VUD preoperatively clearly has a role in deciding when and what surgical procedure should be carried out. Its role in patients after AC is less clearly defined. In cases of urinary incontinence post-AC, with or without upper tract changes, urodynamic studies may be just one tool utilized in the diagnostic effort to clarify the etiology for the suboptimal results of the reconstructed lower urinary tract.

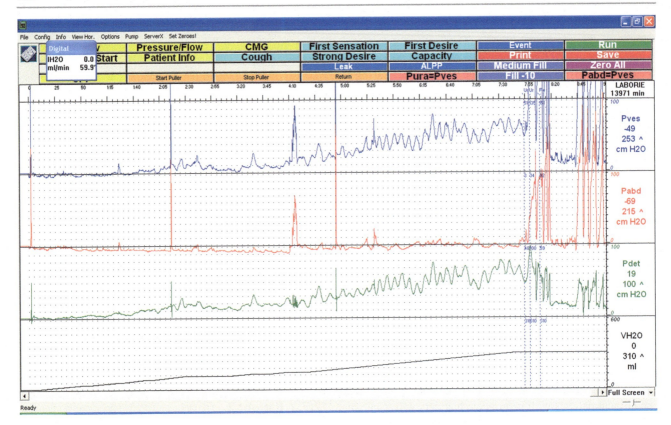

Fig. 12.1 Urodynamic study for Patient 1

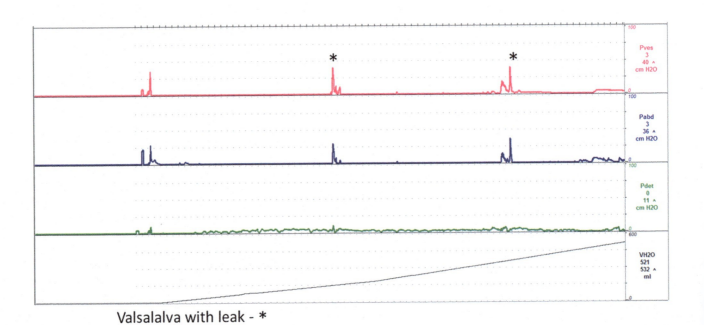

Valsalalva with leak - *

Fig. 12.2 Urodynamic study for Patient 2

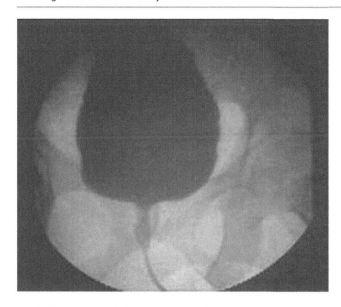

Fig. 12.3 Fluoroscopic image for Patient 2

References

1. Goldmark E, Niver B, Ginsberg DA. Neurogenic bladder: from diagnosis to management. Curr Urol Rep. 2014;15(10):448.
2. McGuire EJ, Woodside JR, Borden TA, Weiss RM. Prognostic value of urodynamic testing in myelodysplastic patients. J Urol. 1981;126(2):205–9.
3. Welk BK, Herschorn S. Augmentation cystoplasty. AUA update series 2012;31: Lesson 20.
4. Greenwell TJ, Venn SN, Mundy AR. Augmentation cystoplasty. BJU Int. 2001;88(6):511–25.
5. Awad SA, Al-Zahrani HM, Gajewski JB, Bourque-Kehoe AA. Long-term results and complications of augmentation ileocystoplasty for idiopathic urge incontinence in women. Br J Urol. 1998;81(4):569–73.
6. Spencer JR, Filmer RB. Malignancy associated with urinary tract reconstruction using enteric segments. Cancer Treat Res. 1992;59:75–87.
7. Veenboer PW, Nadorp S, de Jong TP, Dik P, van Asbeck FW, Bosch JL, de Kort LM. Enterocystoplasty vs detrusorectomy: outcome in the adult with spina bifida. J Urol. 2013;189(3):1066–70.
8. Hansen EL, Hvistendahl GM, Rawashdeh YF, Olsen LH. Promising long-term outcome of bladder autoaugmentation in children with neurogenic bladder dysfunction. J Urol. 2013;190(5):1869–75.
9. Marte A, Di Meglio D, Cotrufo AM, Di Iorio G, De Pasquale M, Vessella A. A long-term follow-up of autoaugmentation in myelodysplastic children. BJU Int. 2002;89(9):928–31.
10. MacNeily AE, Afshar K, Coleman GU, Johnson HW. Autoaugmentation by detrusor myotomy: its lack of effectiveness in the management of congenital neuropathic bladder. J Urol. 2003;170(4 Pt 2):1643–6.
11. Cruz F, Nitti V. Chapter 5: clinical data in neurogenic detrusor overactivity (NDO) and overactive bladder (OAB). Neurourol Urodyn. 2014;33 Suppl 3:S26–31.
12. Ginsberg D, Gousse A, Keppenne V, Sievert KD, Thompson C, Lam W, Brin MF, Jenkins B, Haag-Molkenteller C. Phase 3 efficacy and tolerability study of onabotulinumtoxinA for urinary incontinence from neurogenic detrusor overactivity. J Urol. 2012;187(6):2131–9.
13. Cruz F, Herschorn S, Aliotta P, Brin M, Thompson C, Lam W, Daniell G, Heesakkers J, Haag-Molkenteller C. Efficacy and safety of onabotulinumtoxinA in patients with urinary incontinence due to neurogenic detrusor overactivity: a randomised, double-blind, placebo-controlled trial. Eur Urol. 2011;60(4):742–50.
14. Goldmark E, Benjamin Y, Ginsberg D. Changes in bladder management in patients with neurogenic bladder with FDA approval of onabotulinumtoxina: a reteospective review. Neurourol Urodyn. 2014;33(2):162–266.
15. Biers SM, Venn SN, Greenwell TJ. The past, present and future of augmentation cystoplasty. BJU Int. 2012;109(9):1280–93.
16. Pannek J, Göcking K, Bersch U. Long-term effects of repeated intradetrusor botulinum neurotoxin A injections on detrusor function in patients with neurogenic bladder dysfunction. BJU Int. 2009;104(9):1246–50.
17. Husmann DA. Malignancy after gastrointestinal augmentation in childhood. Ther Adv Urol. 2009;1(1):5–11.
18. Higuchi TT, Granberg CF, Fox JA, Husmann DA. Augmentation cystoplasty and risk of neoplasia: fact, fiction and controversy. J Urol. 2010;184(6):2492–6.
19. Månsson W, Bakke A, Bergman B, Brekkan E, Jonsson O, Kihl B, Nurmi M, Pedersen J, Schultz A, Sørensen B, Urnes T, Wolf H. Perforation of continent urinary reservoirs. Scandinavian experience. Scand J Urol Nephrol. 1997;31(6):529–32.
20. Rosenberg S, Gofrit ON, Hidas G, Landau EH, Pode D. Diagnosing spontaneous ileal neobladder perforation: too often delayed. Can Urol Assoc J. 2013;7(11–12):E817–19.
21. Quek ML, Ginsberg DA. Long-term urodynamics followup of bladder augmentation for neurogenic bladder. J Urol. 2003;169(1):195–8.
22. Herschorn S, Hewitt RJ. Patient perspective of long-term outcome of augmentation cystoplasty for neurogenic bladder. Urology. 1998;52(4):672–8.
23. Seth JH, Haslam C, Panicker JN. Ensuring patient adherence to clean intermittent self-catheterization. Patient Prefer Adherence. 2014;8:191–8.
24. Sekar P, Wallace DD, Waites KB, DeVivo MJ, Lloyd LK, Stover SL, Dubovsky EV. Comparison of long-term renal function after spinal cord injury using different urinary management methods. Arch Phys Med Rehabil. 1997;78(9):992–7.
25. Kaplan SA, Chancellor MB, Blaivas JG. Bladder and sphincter behavior in patients with spinal cord lesions. J Urol. 1991;146(1):113–17.
26. Weld KJ, Dmochowski RR. Association of level of injury and bladder behavior in patients with post-traumatic spinal cord injury. Urology. 2000;55(4):490–4.
27. Wyndaele JJ. Correlation between clinical neurological data and urodynamic function in spinal cord injured patients. Spinal Cord. 1997;35(4):213–16.
28. Watanabe T, Rivas DA, Chancellor MB. Urodynamics of spinal cord injury. Urol Clin North Am. 1996;23(3):459–73.
29. Danforth TL, Ginsberg DA. Neurogenic lower urinary tract dysfunction: how, when, and with which patients do we use urodynamics? Urol Clin North Am. 2014;41(3):445–52.
30. Light K, Cinman A, Giles GR, van Blerk PJ. Urodynamics in congenital neurogenic bladder. S Afr J Surg. 1978;16(4):237–40.
31. McGuire EJ, Woodside JR, Borden TA, Weiss RM. Prognostic value of urodynamic testing in myelodysplastic patients. 1981. J Urol. 2002;167(2 Pt 2):1049–53.
32. Whiteneck GG, Charlifue SW, Frankel HL, Fraser MH, Gardner BP, Gerhart KA, Krishnan KR, Menter RR, Nuseibeh I, Short DJ, et al. Mortality, morbidity, and psychosocial outcomes of persons spinal cord injured more than 20 years ago. Paraplegia. 1992;30(9):617–30.
33. Soden RJ, Walsh J, Middleton JW, Craven ML, Rutkowski SB, Yeo JD. Causes of death after spinal cord injury. Spinal Cord. 2000;38(10):604–10.

34. Chartier-Kastler EJ, Mongiat-Artus P, Bitker MO, Chancellor MB, Richard F, Denys P. Long-term results of augmentation cystoplasty in spinal cord injury. Spinal Cord. 2000;38(8):490–4.
35. Van der Aa F, Joniau S, De Baets K, De Ridder D. Continent catheterizable vesicostomy in an adult population: success at high costs. Neurourol Urodyn. 2009;28(6):487–91.
36. Pope 4th JC, Keating MA, Casale AJ, Rink RC. Augmenting the augmented bladder: treatment of the contractile bowel segment. J Urol. 1998;160(3 Pt 1):854–7.
37. Cher ML, Allen TD. Continence in the myelodysplastic patient following enterocystoplasty. J Urol. 1993;149(5):1103–6.
38. Medel R, Ruarte AC, Herrera M, Castera R, Podesta ML. Urinary continence outcome after augmentation ileocystoplasty as a single surgical procedure in patients with myelodysplasia. J Urol. 2002;168(4 Pt 2):1849–52.
39. McInerney PD, DeSouza N, Thomas PJ, Mundy AR. The role of urodynamic studies in the evaluation of patients with augmentation cystoplasties. Br J Urol. 1995;76(4):475–8.

Adolescent/Early Adult Former Pediatric Neurogenic Patients: Special Considerations

Benjamin Abelson and Hadley M. Wood

13.1 Introduction

The term neurogenic bladder is used to refer to a variety of clinical phenotypes and many unique disease processes—from spinal dysraphism and degenerative neurological disorders to spinal cord injury [1]. For example, Hellstrom and colleagues found varied clinical presentations in patients with tethered cord syndrome and no unifying urological diagnosis or presenting symptom [2]. Patients with tethered cord may present with overactive bladder, changes in bladder capacity, high post-void residual (PVR), underactive bladder, decreased compliance, or detrusor sphincter dyssynergia (DSD) [3]. As a diagnosis, "neurogenic bladder" does not imply a uniform treatment modality, and in fact, patients with the diagnosis may be best served by drastically different therapies, including behavior modification, pharmacotherapy, or urogenital reconstruction. Given our understanding of the complex neuroanatomical pathways involved in micturition, one could expect that a neurological "find the lesion" methodology could cleanly categorize phenotypes. However, texts that have utilized this approach demonstrate the variability in symptoms, urodynamic studies, and treatment response in patients with lesions "above the brainstem" or at certain spinal cord levels [4].

Given the variability in clinical presentation of patients with similar mechanisms of neurological dysfunction, a neurological examination is insufficient in therapeutic decision-making for patients with neurogenic dysfunction of the lower urinary tract. For example, Wyndaele and colleagues evaluated 92 patients with traumatic spinal cord injury in order to determine the diagnostic relevance of clinical criteria in regard to lower urinary tract function [5]. Although they do demonstrate a correlation between neuroanatomical pathways and clinical symptoms—i.e., patients with lesions above T10 typically have poor compliance and detrusor overactivity—the authors recognize that variability in presentation makes urodynamic evaluation crucial to guiding treatment decisions. The authors attribute this variability to coexisting subclinical lesions, variability in cord-column correlation, damage to detrusor muscle from overdistention, or absent/reduced reflexes in patients with normal neuroanatomy.

Recognizing the incomplete clinical relevance of neurological evaluation has made urodynamic studies (UDS) central to diagnosis, categorization, management, and surveillance of patients with a congenitally abnormal lower urinary tract. Urodynamic testing gives providers a tool with which we can make diagnoses, identify treatment options, and monitor treatment response. Perhaps more importantly, urodynamics allow for identification of patients at risk of upper urinary tract deterioration [6].

One of the most effective examples of utilizing UDS to categorize patients with neurogenic dysfunction is described for patients being followed after fetal myelomeningocele repair [7]. Since the MOMS trial demonstrated that prenatal myelomeningocele repair decreases the need for ventriculoperitoneal shunting and improves motor and cognitive scores compared to patients treated postnatally, we can now begin to understand the urological outcomes of patients with prenatal repair [8]. Leal da Cruz and colleagues characterized 51 patients who underwent prenatal myelomeningocele repair into four categories:

1. Normal: Stable bladder cystometry without leakage
2. High risk: Overactive bladder with detrusor leak point higher than 40 cm H_2O
3. Incontinent: Overactive bladder with detrusor leak point pressure lower than 40 cm H_2O or stable bladder with leaking below 40 cm H_2O
4. Underactivity: Underactive bladder with high PVR

B. Abelson, M.D. • H.M. Wood, M.D., F.A.C.S. (✉)
Glickman Urological and Kidney Institute
Department of Urology, Cleveland Clinic,
9500 Euclid Avenue, Q10, Cleveland, OH 44195, USA
e-mail: abelsob@ccf.org; woodh@ccf.org

Such categorization allowed for development of a clear treatment algorithm in which patients in the normal or incontinent groups underwent surveillance, patients in the high-risk group were treated with clean intermittent catheterization (CIC) and anticholinergic medication, and patients in the underactivity group were treated with CIC alone [7].

Part of the challenge of categorizing patients with neurogenic bladder is that the neuromuscular physiology of micturition is dynamic, and a certain phenotype cannot describe a patient from the in utero period through adulthood. Furthermore, as patients with neurological diseases associated with voiding dysfunction live longer, we are presented with the complexity of long-term physiologic changes (i.e., BPH, prolapse) [9]. In addition, innovations in neurosurgical, reconstructive, and fetal interventions are generating a new patient population with unique urological presentations [8].

The goal of this chapter is to describe three major phenotypes of patients who have congenitally abnormal lower urinary tracts. We will present the detailed clinical questions that need to be asked in order to fully assess each index patient's symptoms and the clinical workup necessary to assist in categorizing each patient. Then we will discuss several patient cases that represent each phenotype. Although treatment is not the focus of this chapter, we will also briefly introduce the treatment modalities that are implicated for each patient phenotype. Lastly, we discuss considerations for renal transplantation.

13.2 Clinical Evaluation

The clinical history can provide invaluable clues toward reaching a diagnosis and establishing treatment goals when evaluating a patient with neurogenic lower urinary tract dysfunction. What is the chief complaint: leakage, obstructive voiding symptoms, recurrent infection, or frequency? Is the primary reason for the visit concern for the upper tracts or patient symptoms? Are the symptoms progressive or stable? Did they begin acutely? Does the patient suffer from frequency at night or during the day? Is the patient a positional voider? Relevant review of systems must also include bowel function and habits, other medical comorbidities (e.g., sleep apnea in the myelomeningocele population, which promotes nocturnal polyuria), and a complete neurological history. Understanding the temporal patterns of the patient's other neurological sequelae may also help the provider develop a better understanding of the stability of the patient's urological disease.

A voiding diary is an essential component to the history and physical exam in a patient with neurogenic bladder. It not only assists in diagnosis, but it can help gauge the efficacy of treatment. In addition to a complete review of medical and surgical history, review of systems, physical exam, and social and family history, initial evaluation should include, at a minimum, a urinalysis and post-void residual (in those voiding). Additional evaluation, including upper tract and bladder/reservoir imaging (ultrasound or computed tomography), serum studies (creatinine), and renal functional investigation (nuclear renal scan, 24 h urine collection, or others), may also be warranted. It must be noted that particularly in the non weight-bearing adult myelomeningocele population, there remains no well-defined gold standard for estimation of GFR. We have demonstrated that creatinine-based techniques (MDRD, Cockroft-Gault, 24 h urine) are inaccurate [10]. Cystatin and iothalamate renal scanning, while initially promising, have limitations as well.

While the classic approach to pediatric urologic care is very close monitoring in infancy and young childhood with regular, but less intensive, follow-up after the bladder has "declared" itself, renal deterioration is well described during periadolescence. The reasons for this are likely multifactorial, but most point to rapid skeletal growth and poorer compliance ("teenage rebellion") as the most likely contributors. High-grade reflux, female gender, and initiation of CIC at a later age are suggested as the most important risk factors for renal deterioration in this population [11]. Nevertheless, regular monitoring is absolutely mandatory during this period. De Kort and colleagues suggest annual urodynamic testing while the patient is still growing and then only as indicated by new symptoms or new ultrasound findings in those who have completed growth [12]. This is probably a reasonable approach as long as close surveillance and regular, thorough histories are taken with each visit until prospective studies and a consensus panel are able to better define surveillance guidelines. In addition, during this period, patients should be prepared for transition to adult care providers, a process that often requires close and frequent office visits.

13.3 Case Studies

13.3.1 Type 1: Classic Neurogenic Bladder

Presenting symptom: Classic neurogenic bladder is most often characterized by a small-capacity, overactive bladder that demonstrates poor compliance. As such, presenting symptoms can vary. The most obvious and most common presentation is progressive and bothersome leakage or a shortened dry interval between CIC. Long-term sequelae of leakage, like skin breakdown or urethral fistulae secondary to indwelling catheters, may also be a presenting symptom of neurogenic bladder. Other patients present with increasing frequency or recurrent UTI or pyelonephritis. This is a particularly worrisome finding, as it may suggest development of secondary reflux which carries risk of renal scarring. Tethered cord has been associated with periods of linear growth or can be seen later in adulthood with progressive disc disease and spinal stenosis. This may present with or without urological symptoms, in addition to lower extremity weakness, loss of coordination, ulcers, burns, or worsened bowel dysfunction. Even more distressing is that this condition may develop without any obvious symptoms such that the first sign may be new hydronephrosis seen on screening ultrasound or rising serum creatinine on annual lab work. The later scenario demonstrates why surveillance with history, physical exam, and noninvasive testing is so crucial.

13.3.2 Patient 1: T.R.

13.3.2.1 History
T.R. is a 24-year-old man with a history of myelomeningocele at birth who was managed with timed voiding and anticholinergics and was followed closely through childhood. Around age 18, he noted lower extremity weakness and underwent spinal surgery to address tether. Urodynamics shortly after surgery demonstrated a weak bladder with elevated PVR (100 cm^3), and the patient was instructed on intermittent catheterization and continued anticholinergics. T.R. discontinued follow-up in pediatric myelomeningocele clinic shortly thereafter, given his age. He returned to an adult clinic 6 years later with an increasingly shortened dry interval (now about 2 h) and nighttime bedwetting.

13.3.2.2 Physical Examination
General: Normal body habitus, walks without assist devices with slight foot drop
Cardiac: Regular rate and rhythm, no murmurs, rubs, or gallops
Pulmonary: Chest clear to auscultation without wheezing, rales, or rhonchi
Neurological: No sensation to touch in penile shaft or perineum, atonic lower extremities
Abdominal: Soft, non-tender, non-distended, no masses
Genitourinary: Normal external genitalia other than sensation as noted above
Psychiatric: Normal mood and affect

13.3.2.3 Lab Work/Other Studies
BUN/Cr = 11/0.76
Renal ultrasound revealed non-hydronephrotic kidneys (11.2 and 10.5 cm in length) with a thick-walled bladder with significant internal debris.

13.3.2.4 UDS

Findings
Filling
The patient was filled to a maximum capacity of 148 cm^3, with first sensation at 57 cm^3 and strong desire at 96 cm^3. The maximum filling detrusor pressure was 40 cm of water. There was a steady rise of Pdet during filling.

Voiding
The patient voluntarily voided 140 cm^3 with Valsalva, and the urethral catheter needed to be removed to allow for complete emptying. The patient did not empty completely, with a Pdet Q max of 35 cm^3 H$_2$O, maximum flow of 7 cm^3/s, and catheterized PVR of 120 cm^3.

Impression
Videourodynamic studies demonstrate a small-capacity (<150 cm^3) bladder that was poorly compliant, as evidenced by a storage pressure around 47 mmHg at capacity (Fig. 13.1a). The video images demonstrate classic "Christmas tree" appearance (Fig. 13.1b). No secondary reflux was seen, although AP images typical of most VUDS often fail to demonstrate low-grade reflux, as the refluxing ureters are hidden by the full bladder.

13.3.2.5 Treatment Options
Patients in this category typically have small-capacity bladders with poor compliance and detrusor overactivity. Treatment options include anticholinergics, augmentation, or Botox. In this case, this patient was already on anticholinergics, and the severity of bladder wall changes demonstrated by VUDS and ultrasound often suggest poor prognosis with Botox alone. However, the patient was in college and opted for Botox injections prior to proceeding with surgical management. He has Crohn's disease, and therefore any bowel operation presents additional risk of postoperative complications, not to mention activation of disease in the augmentation cystoplasty. Autoaugmentation has not proven to be durable in this situation, and bladder substitutes (tissue-engineered bladder) are presently investigational.

13.3.3 Type 2: Hypotonic/Atonic Bladder (With or Without Detrusor Overactivity)

Presenting symptom: A hypotonic or atonic bladder is less commonly seen in patients with myelomeningocele, but often observed in older patients with a history of posterior urethral valves, dysfunctional voiding, cerebral palsy, and congenital neuromuscular disease. Patients typically present with infrequent, large-volume voids. In the case of adults with cerebral palsy, large-volume episodes of enuresis occurring once or twice daily or worsening urinary tract infections are classically reported. While it is distressing to not intervene in such circumstances with initiation of CIC, it is important to note that CIC in many of these patients is quite troublesome and not without risk. For patients with PUV, catheterization can be difficult owing to dilation of the posterior urethra and the classic high bladder neck that these patients often have. Patients with cerebral palsy, neuromuscular disease, and myelomeningocele often have lower

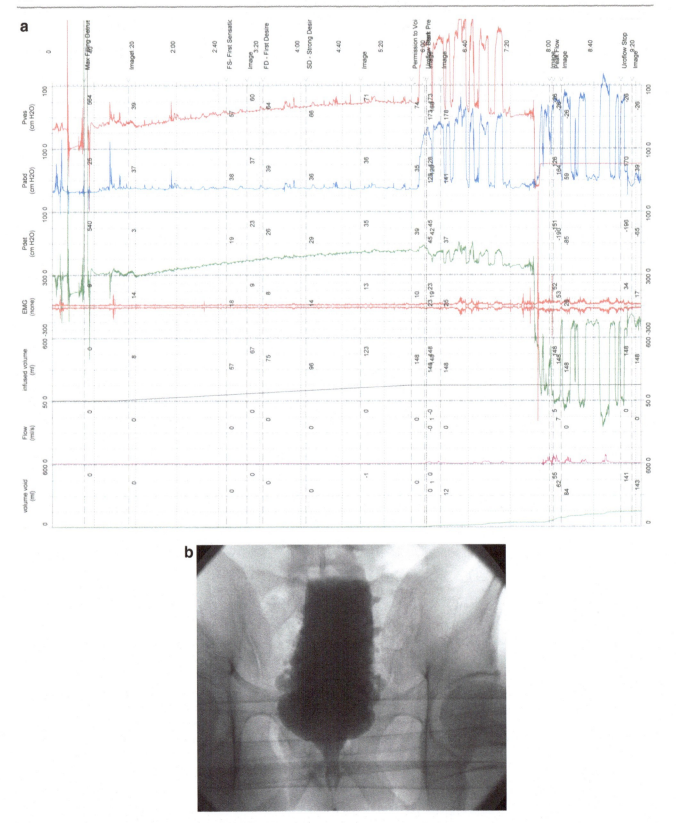

Fig. 13.1 (**a, b**) T.R. is a 24-year-old man with myelomeningocele status post tether release at 18 years who was lost to follow-up for 6 years then presented to adult clinic with frequency and nocturnal enuresis; (**a**) urodynamics demonstrating a small-capacity bladder with poor compliance; (**b**) classic "Christmas tree" bladder

extremity contractures and anatomy that makes catheterization very challenging, not to mention that as adults they often do not have reliable and consistent assistance if impaired manual dexterity makes self-catheterization difficult. If technical or social challenges mean that the patient is only able to successfully catheterize every 1–2 days, risk of UTI may actually increase due to reinoculation of the bladder with each introduction of a catheter. For these reasons, characterization of the bladder storage pressures is critical. Even near 1 L capacity, many of these bladders demonstrate storage pressures at 10 mmHg or below and no reflux.

13.3.4 Patient 2: M.E.

13.3.4.1 History
M.E. is a 44-year-old male born with myelomeningocele. In childhood he was ambulatory and performed CIC about every 3 h and was maintained on anticholinergics. Around age 20, he was in a car accident and sustained a closed head injury which left him wheelchair bound without consistent urological care. He presented to adult myelomeningocele clinic at age 44 with a complaint of incontinence leading to ulcers on his legs and buttocks and erectile dysfunction. He reported no use of anticholinergics and Valsalva voided every 3 h with leakage in between (noted most often when transferring in and out of his chair).

13.3.4.2 Physical Examination
General: Obese, in wheelchair, no acute distress
Cardiac: Regular rate and rhythm, no murmurs, rubs, or gallops
Pulmonary: Chest clear to auscultation without wheezing, rales, or rhonchi
Neurological: Paraplegia
Abdominal Soft, non-tender, non-distended, no masses. RLQ scar well healed
Genitourinary: Normal external genitalia, atonic lower extremities, and central obesity
Psychiatric: No signs of depression, anxiety, or agitation

13.3.4.3 Lab Work/Other Studies
BUN/Cr = 13/0.8
Renal ultrasound demonstrated 12 cm and 11.7 cm kidneys without hydronephrosis.

13.3.4.4 UDS

Findings

Filling
The bladder was filled to a capacity of about 550 cm^3, with first sensation at 75 cm^3, strong desire at 221 cm^3, and permission to void at 516 cm^3. The bladder demonstrated good compliance and no detrusor overactivity, with maximum filling detrusor pressure of 14 cm H$_2$O. The patient leaked during stress maneuvers during filling with a leak point pressure of 78 cm H$_2$O.

Voiding
The patient voided to completion with Valsalva. Maximum detrusor pressure with Valsalva was 160 cm H$_2$O with Pdet Qmax of 43 cm H$_2$O. Flow rate was unable to be recorded as the patient could not void into the funnel.

Impression
Videourodynamics revealed a large smooth-walled, compliant, and stable bladder that emptied to completion with Valsalva, though the patient leaked with stress maneuvers (Fig. 13.2a–c).

13.3.4.5 Treatment Options
See next section.

13.3.5 Patient 3: B.R.

13.3.5.1 History
B.R. is a 56-year-old female with history of cerebral palsy, managed with Crede voiding her entire life. In general, she had experienced approximately two nonfebrile UTIs per year. She voids about five times during the day and once at night. She was referred by another urologist for "slowly rising creatinine, mild bilateral pelvicaliectasis, prevoid volume of 732 cm^3, and post-void volume 277 cm^3."

13.3.5.2 Physical Examination
General: Contracted lower extremities, well nourished
Cardiac: Regular rate and rhythm, no murmurs, rubs, or gallops
Pulmonary: Chest clear to auscultation, no wheezes, rubs, or rhonchi
Neurological: Severe lower extremity contractures
Abdominal: Soft, non-tender, non-distended, no masses
Genitourinary: Pelvic exam deferred
Psychiatric: Anxious, impaired cognition

13.3.5.3 Lab Work/Other Studies
Cr = 1.14 (2012)
Cr = 1.31 (2015)

13.3.5.4 UDS

Findings
Filling
The bladder was filled to a capacity of 700 cm^3, with no first sensation or feeling of coolness, strong desire at 590 cm^3, and permission to void at 600 cm^3. The bladder demonstrated

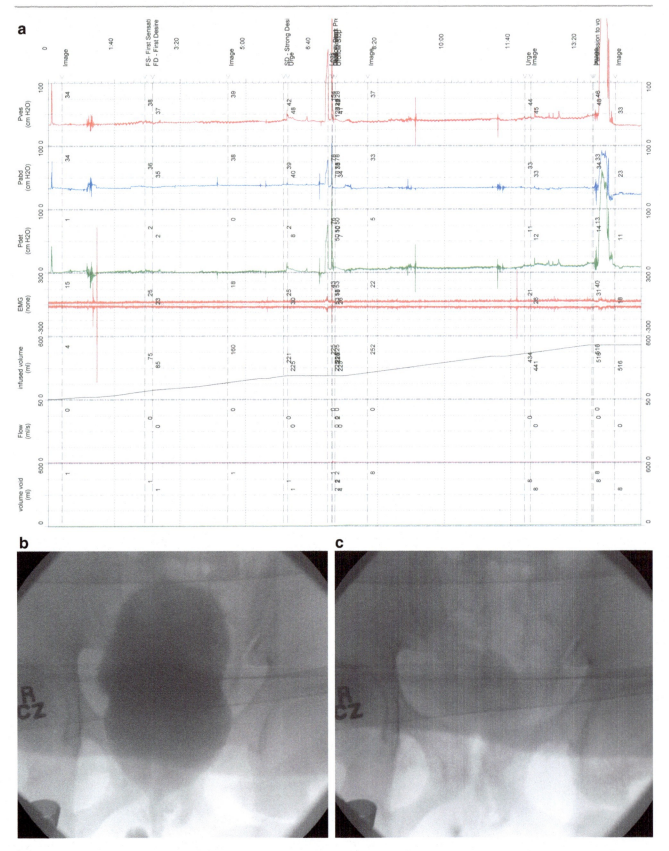

Fig. 13.2 (**a–c**) M.E. is a 44-year-old man with history of myelomeningocele followed by motor vehicle accident and head injury at age 20. He presented at age 44 with incontinence and Valsalva voiding; (**a**) urodynamics demonstrating large-capacity bladder that was smooth walled with maximal storage pressure of 12 mmHg at 516 cm^3; (**b**) filling; (**c**) post void

good compliance and no detrusor overactivity, with maximum filling detrusor pressure of 4 cm H$_2$O. The patient had no leakage with stress maneuvers.

Voiding

The patient was unable to void with catheters in place but voided 350 cm^3 on uroflow with a maximum flow of 33 mL/s. Maximum detrusor pressure with straining was 15 cm H$_2$O. Her post-void residual was approximately 350 cm^3.

Impression

Urodynamics demonstrated a compliant bladder with a capacity around 700 cm^3, no leakage, and a post-void residual after straining to void of 350 cm^3.

See Fig. 13.3.

13.3.5.5 Treatment Options

Both patients 2 and 3 have low-pressure, weak bladders with minimal detrusor overactivity. Terminal DO is often present in patients with cerebral palsy, and phasic DO can be seen in patients with several different underlying etiologies. Cognitive state and the status of the bladder outlet often drive management for symptomatic DO. In both of these cases, neither patient demonstrated DO on UDS or clinical evaluation. Patient 2 (M.E.) was distressed by his leakage and had already had significant sequelae (skin breakdown) related to incontinence. Artificial urinary sphincter is used in the management of bladder neck incompetence for many individuals with myelomeningocele; although for those using CIC, we typically recommend it be placed at the bladder neck to minimize the risk of urethral erosion. This operation can be quite technically challenging and potentially morbid in an adult with myelomeningocele, particularly if he mobilizes via wheelchair and is obese. Fortunately for patient 2, he is able to empty entirely and quite quickly by Valsalva and is an excellent candidate for a bulbar urethral AUS. Patient 3 demonstrated limited baseline cognitive function and severe lower extremity contractures. Moreover, she was being cared for by her adult sibling who worked outside the home and depended on home care aides and

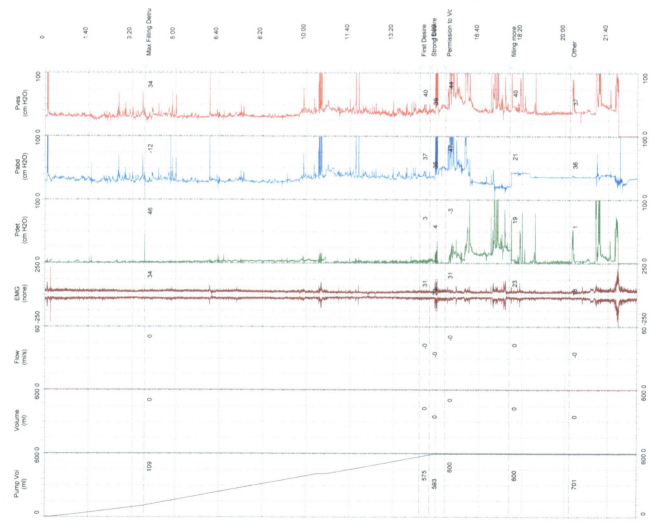

Fig. 13.3 B.R. is a 56-year-old woman with a history of cerebral palsy, managed with Crede voiding her entire life. She was referred to us for gradual increase in creatinine, mild bilateral pelvicaliectasis, and PVR of about 300 cm^3. UDS revealed no leak with stress and a stable, compliant bladder through filling to 600 cm^3. PVR was 350 cm^3 after she voided 346 cm^3 after the catheters were removed

friends during the working hours, which precluded reliable intermittent catheterization. Due to these factors, CIC was not a sustainable option. The patient underwent suprapubic tube placement after serial creatinine demonstrated progression of chronic kidney disease.

13.3.6 Type 3: DSD, Neurogenic

Detrusor sphincter dyssynergia can coexist with any bladder phenotype. It is critical to establish whether it is present, as treatment involves sphincterotomy or botulinum A injection into the sphincter and in some scenarios, may convert a partially continent patient to entirely continent, or prevent the need for intermittent catheterization. Suggestions that DSD may be present on clinical history include straining and positional voiding, Crede voiding, and/or voiding in a staccato pattern. It is our practice to utilize videourodynamics in all situations where DSD is entertained, since patch EMG is insensitive. The classic finding is a dilated posterior urethra and non-opening or poor opening of the sphincter and a staccato pattern on uroflow.

13.3.7 Patient 4: J.G.

13.3.7.1 History
J.G. is a 20-year-old with myelomeningocele who was managing his bladder with timed voiding and CIC twice daily on bactrim prophylaxis and anticholinergics. He experienced very few problems for several years on this regimen. The rationale for twice daily CIC did not make a lot of medical sense, but had worked well for him. We made a plan to wean CIC to once daily and then discontinue altogether and follow his renal ultrasounds, Cr, and symptoms. Over the next couple of years, his creatinine slowly increased, which prompted urodynamic studies.

13.3.7.2 Physical Examination
General: Central obesity, walks with braces on both legs
Cardiac: Regular rate and rhythm, no murmurs, rubs, or gallops
Pulmonary: Clear to auscultation, no wheezes, rales, or rhonchi
Neurological: Normal cognition, full ROM and function of UEs, weak LEs
Abdominal: Non-tender, no masses
Genitourinary: Normal external genitalia
Psychiatric: Normal mood and affect

13.3.7.3 Lab Work/Other Studies
Cr = 0.84 (2011)
Cr = 1.06 (2015)
Renal ultrasound revealed kidneys of 10.9 and 11.5 cm without hydronephrosis.

13.3.7.4 UDS

Findings

Filling
The bladder was filled to a capacity of 245 cm^3, with strong desire at 224 cm^3. Compliance remained stable throughout most of filling.

Voiding
Voiding was assisted by terminal DO. There was no leakage with urge or stress. The external sphincter did not open over three runs of filling and voiding and PVR remained elevated for each.

Impression
Urodynamics demonstrated detrusor sphincter dyssynergia with small functional bladder capacity.

13.3.7.5 Treatment Options
Videourodynamic studies revealed DSD without opening of the external urinary sphincter (Fig. 13.4a, b). Given his increasing creatinine and elevated post-void residual, we discussed the options including continued observation versus Botox injection in the external urinary sphincter. The patient elected to pursue Botox injections. He underwent injection of 200 U Botox to the external urinary sphincter. Unfortunately the patient did not experience significant improvement in his voiding and complained of small-volume insensate leakage; therefore, he elected to not pursue repeat injection. We will continue to observe him with laboratory studies and ultrasound.

13.3.8 Preparation for Transplant Evaluation

The patient who presents in adult life for renal transplant with neuropathic bladder is poorly described, and sorting out how one deals with both the bladder and the often hydronephrotic, poorly draining native kidneys can indeed be challenging. Part of that challenge rests in understanding what the patient's goals are for continence postoperatively, and part requires very good communication with the transplant team to understand what their concerns are related to anatomy in an often multiply operated abdomen.

13.3.9 Patient 5: T.O.

13.3.9.1 History
T.O. is a 35-year-old man with a history of posterior urethral valves who had bilateral ureterostomies during infancy followed by re-anastomosis at age 3. He began having recurrent UTIs and nocturnal enuresis as a teenager, developed hypertension in his twenties, and underwent right nephrectomy. He

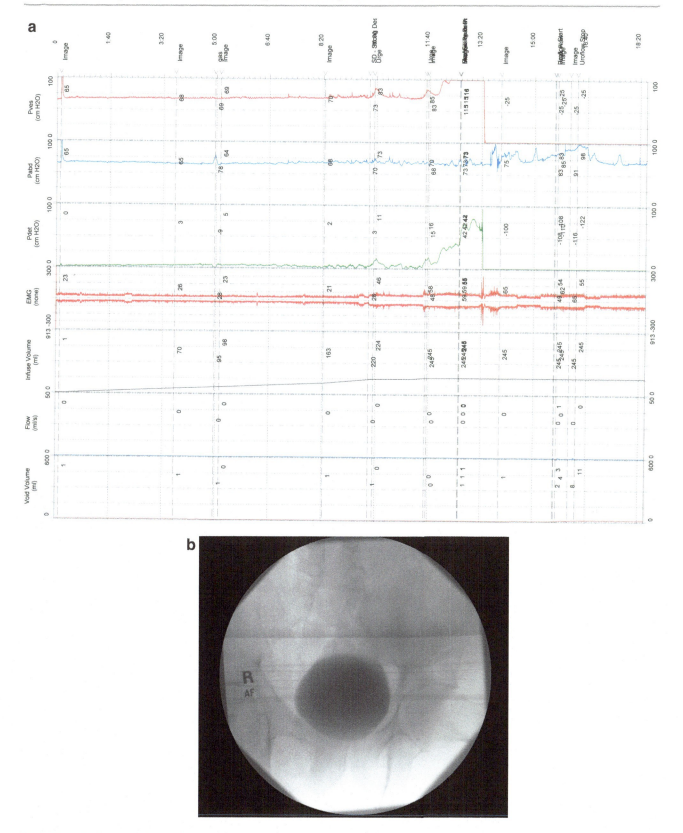

Fig. 13.4 (**a**, **b**) J.G. is a 20-year-old with myelomeningocele who was managing his bladder with timed voiding and CIC twice daily on Bactrim prophylaxis and anticholinergics who was found to have a small-capacity bladder and DSD (**a**) without opening of the external urinary sphincter (**b**)

was referred with severe renal insufficiency and an inability to perform intermittent catheterization owing to posterior urethral dilation and pain with catheterization. His renal function had deteriorated and he was getting recurrent UTIs from infrequent catheterization and incomplete Valsalva voiding.

13.3.9.2 Physical Examination

General: No deformities, normal nutrition, healthy appearing
Cardiac: Regular rate and rhythm, no murmurs, rubs, or gallops
Pulmonary: Chest clear to auscultation without wheezing, rales, or rhonchi
Neurological: Grossly normal motor and sensory function
Abdominal: Suprapubic scar and bilateral ureterostomy scars, well healed
Genitourinary: Descended testicles, orthotopic meatus, 14 Fr Foley catheter in place
Psychiatric: No depression or anxiety

13.3.9.3 Lab Work/Other Studies

GFR was estimated to be 35 and he had a solitary kidney as demonstrated on CT scan.

13.3.9.4 UDS

Finding

Filling

The bladder was filled to a capacity of about 289 cm^3, with first sensation at 149 cm^3 and strong desire at 288 cm^3. Maximum filling detrusor pressure was 30 cm H$_2$O, though the trend of the curve demonstrates his pressures are likely above 40 cm H$_2$O at his typical volumes of 500–700 cm^3. The patient did not leak during stress maneuvers.

Voiding

The patient could not void with catheters in place, though he emptied complete at the conclusion of the study as confirmed by fluoroscopy.

Cystoscopy

The anterior urethra was normal and the posterior urethral consistent with prior valve ablation. The prostate was high riding with a dilated prostatic fossa, and the patient's bladder was massively trabeculated with a "Christmas tree" appearance.

Impression

Urodynamics demonstrate a poorly compliant and small-capacity bladder and paired with the cystoscopic findings suggest high-pressure end-stage neurogenic bladder.
See Fig. 13.5a.

13.3.9.5 Treatment Options

While many bladder phenotypes can be seen for adults with posterior urethral valves, this patient demonstrated a poorly compliant, small-capacity bladder. He was unable to void on pressure flow studies but voided completely with Valsalva maneuvers after the catheter was removed, suggesting high voiding pressures as well. Both incontinent diversion (ileal conduit) and augmentation cystoplasty with catheterizable channel were offered, the former being suggested as the option with the best possibility for delaying renal replacement. However, the patient adamantly refused incontinent diversion, electing for augmentation cystoplasty with appendicovesicostomy (Fig. 13.5b–e).

He is quite polyuric (he makes about 7 L of urine daily) and has diabetes insipidus related to his renal insufficiency which impairs his ability to have a reasonable dry interval, even with a bladder capacity after augmentation of over 500 cm^3. For that reason, he places a catheter at bedtime for continuous drainage to allow for sleep and to preserve renal function. Two years after surgery, he remains at a GFR near 30 and is therefore not yet listed for transplant.

13.3.10 Patient 6: H.R.

13.3.10.1 History

H.R. is a 47-year-old born with classic bladder exstrophy who underwent multiple operations in childhood (over 15 abdominal exploratory laparotomies), ultimately leaving him with an open bladder neck and augmented bladder. While there were attempts to get him continent, this was never achieved. At the time of evaluation, he was wearing eight heavy pads per day.

13.3.10.2 Physical Examination

General: Within normal limits nutrition, no deformities, healthy appearing
Cardiac: Regular rate and rhythm, no murmurs, rubs, or gallops
Pulmonary: Chest clear to auscultation without wheezes, rales, or rhonchi
Neurological: No gross motor or sensory deficits
Abdominal: Multiple scars from prior surgeries. Pubic diastasis. Penis c/w exstrophy repair in the fashion of Cantwell-Ransley (although known as skin graft extension) with a dorsal location. Visible leakage with palpation of saccular urethra
Genitourinary: Normal external genitalia, atonic lower extremities, and central obesity
Psychiatric: No signs of depression or anxiety

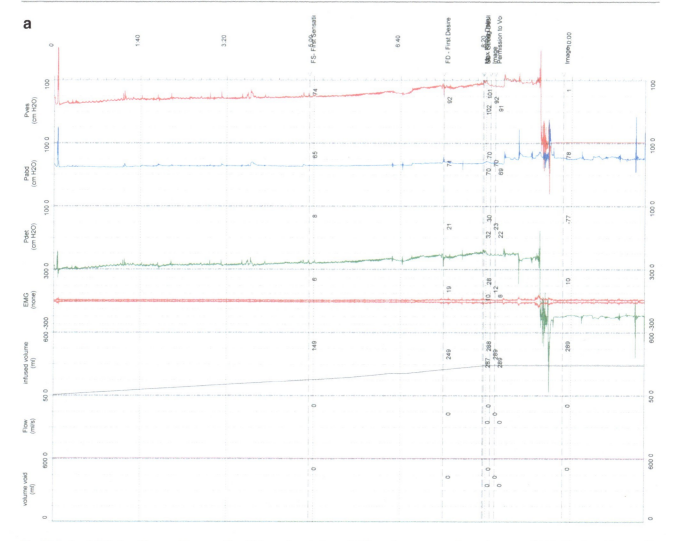

Fig. 13.5 (**a–e**) T.O. is a 37-year-old man with a history of posterior urethral valves and chronic kidney disease, with an inability to catheterize due to valves. He had a poorly compliant, small-capacity bladder. (**a**) He underwent appendicovesicostomy, (**b**) bladder flap, (**c**) appendix mobilized, (**d**) small bowel anastomosed to posterior bladder wall and appendix tunneled, (**e**) postoperative cystogram

13.3.10.3 Lab Work/Other Studies

Creatinine was 5.19 with estimated GFR of 12. CT scan demonstrated bilateral renal parenchymal atrophy with wall thickening and edema of the renal collecting systems and ureters.

13.3.10.4 UDS

Findings
Filling
The bladder was filled to a capacity of about 215 cm^3, with first sensation at 20 cm^3 and strong desire at 191 cm^3. The bladder demonstrated maximum filling detrusor pressure of 23 cm H_2O with urge as well as detrusor overactivity. The patient leaked with Valsalva with leak point pressure of 68 cm H_2O.

Voiding
The patient voided 203 cm^3 involuntarily, with maximum voiding detrusor pressure 15 cm H_2O with straining. His Pdet Q max was 9 cm H_2O with maximum flow rate of 8 cm^3/s.

Impression
Urodynamics demonstrates a small-capacity bladder with leakage associated with both urge and stress and a very low abdominal leak point pressure. The patient Valsalva voids with good emptying.

13.3.10.5 Treatment Options

Urodynamics suggested Valsalva voiding to near completion and leakage with both stress and urge, suggesting that continence would be unlikely to be achieved without bladder neck

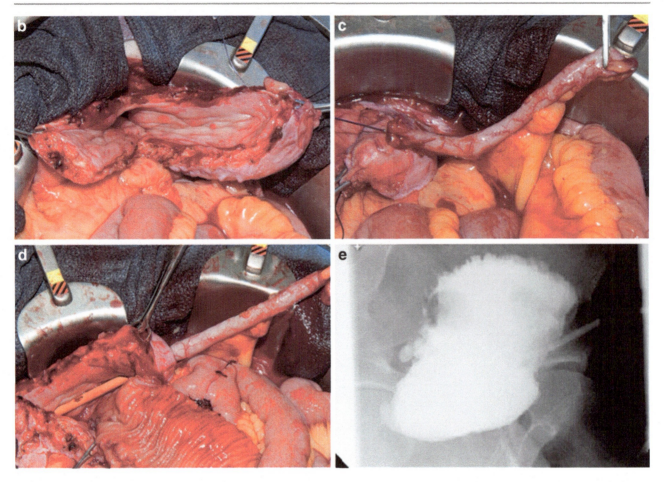

Fig. 13.5 (continued)

sphincter, reconstruction, or closure (Fig. 13.6a). As his urethra does not permit catheterization, alternative methods of bladder emptying were entertained. His CT demonstrates very atrophic hydronephrotic kidneys (Fig. 13.6b), and a cystogram demonstrates a tubular augmented pouch (Fig. 13.6c). VCUG confirmed near-complete emptying with Valsalva. Two issues were of concern in preparation for transplant: First, the native kidneys would always present an opportunity for recurrent infection and would likely need to be removed; and second, achieving continence (if a priority for the patient) would require bladder neck closure and continent catheterizable channel. After discussion about the goals of treatment with the patient, a determination was made to prepare the bladder for continent diversion with subsequent planned living donor transplant. Bladder neck closure with cutaneous ureterostomy and right nephrectomy would initially be performed approximately 6 weeks prior to planned living donor transplant. The new graft would be implanted into the left native renal fossa, and the native left kidney is removed, obviating the need for transabdominal surgery at the time of transplant.

13.3.11 Patient 7: Y.G.

13.3.11.1 History

Y.G. is a 22-year-old man with a history of Eagle-Barrett syndrome status post abdominoplasty, with Mitrofanoff procedure and colostomy performed as an infant. He has one atrophic kidney, had not had prior bladder augmentations, and was diagnosed with VACTERL syndrome. He was managed with CIC four times daily, with 500–750 cm^3 per catheterization.

13.3.11.2 Physical Examination

General: No acute distress
Cardiac: Regular rate and rhythm, no murmurs, rubs, or gallops
Pulmonary: Chest clear to auscultation without wheezes, rales, or rhonchi
Neurological: No gross deficits
Abdominal: Lax abdomen, colostomy pouched on the left abdomen, Mitrofanoff in the right abdomen without evidence of stricture

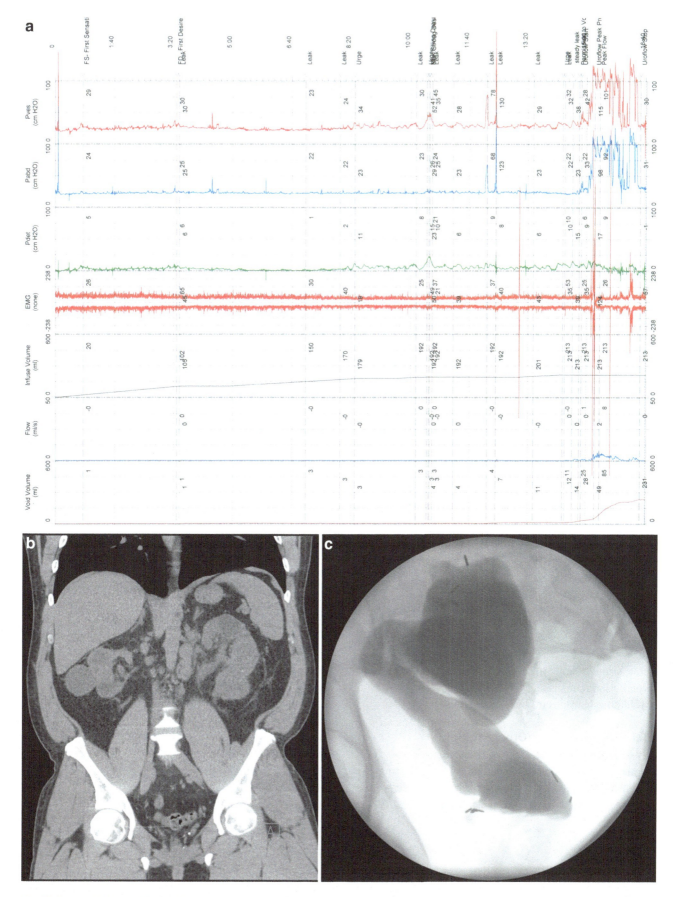

Fig. 13.6 (**a**–**c**) H.R. is a 47-year-old man born with bladder exstrophy who underwent multiple surgeries during childhood which left him with an open bladder neck and augmented bladder; (**a**) UDS demonstrated Valsalva voiding to near completion; (**b**) CT demonstrates very atrophic hydronephrotic kidneys; (**c**) cystogram demonstrates a tubular augmented pouch

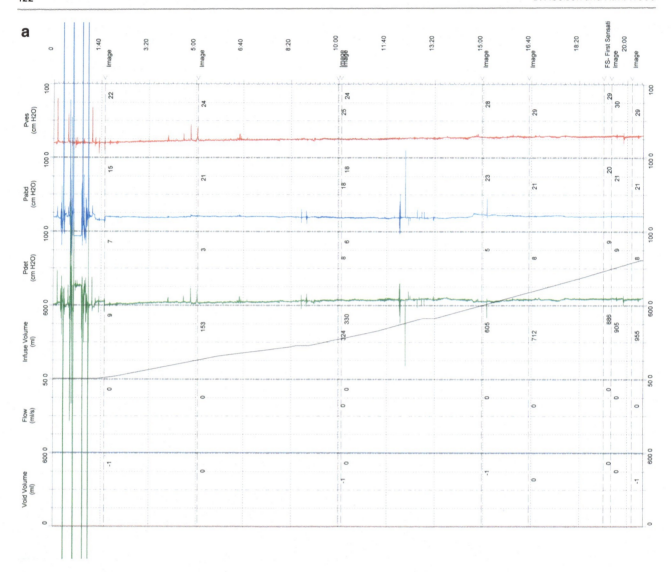

Fig. 13.7 (**a–c**) Y.G. is a 22-year-old man with a history of Eagle-Barrett syndrome status postabdominoplasty with Mitrofanoff procedure and colostomy. UDS demonstrated filling to 1 L and storage at low pressure (**a**) without reflux (**b**). CT demonstrated a thick-walled bladder, dilated ureters, and heavily scarred kidneys (**c**)

Genitourinary: Small right testicle, normal left testicle, small phallus, circumcised

Psychiatric: No signs of depression or anxiety

13.3.11.3 Lab Work/Other Studies

Cr = 4.0, increased from 2.0 two years prior.

Imaging: CT demonstrated bilateral renal scarring with dilated ureters and a markedly thickened bladder wall.

13.3.11.4 UDS

Findings
Filling

The patient was filled to a maximum capacity of 955 cm^3, with first sensation at 886 cm^3 and strong desire at 955 cm^3. Maximum filling detrusor pressure was 9 cm H$_2$O. There was no detrusor overactivity associated with urge or leakage and the patient did not leak when stressed.

Voiding

The patient was unable to void with catheters in place. He was catheterized for 955 cm^3.

Impression

Videourodynamics demonstrated a large-capacity, low-pressure, stable bladder without obvious reflux.

13.3.11.5 Treatment Options

UDS demonstrated filling to 1 L and storage at low pressure without reflux (Fig. 13.7a, b). He underwent CT scan which demonstrated a large, thick-walled bladder and dilated ureters and heavily scarred kidneys with parenchymal loss

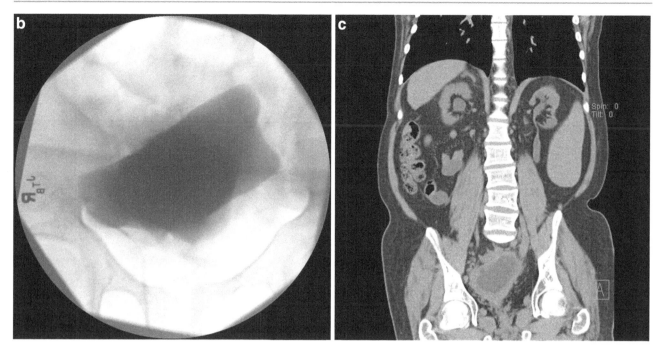

Fig. 13.7 (continued)

(Fig. 13.7c). Given these findings, we felt that his bladder would be safe for transplant but that the kidneys may be a source of infection once immunosuppressed and that bilateral nephrectomies may be needed subsequently. A retroperitoneal approach with placement of his graft in the native left renal fossa and native nephrectomy was determined to be the best initial step, as this would avoid abdominal laparotomy and remove a potential source of infection. His eGFR is near 20, and therefore he has been referred for renal transplantation evaluation.

13.4 Conclusion

Congenital neurogenic bladder is a "catch-all" term that includes patients with diverse phenotypes that require varied interventions. Urodynamics is a crucial tool for diagnosing and monitoring these patients and is indicated in patients with changing urinary symptoms, increased frequency of infections, hematuria, increase serum creatinine, or new upper tract findings. Treatment should be tailored to the individual urodynamic findings and their implications on bladder hostility and long-term renal protection. Continuity from pediatric to adult clinics is critical to providing effective urological care given the unpredictable natural history of bladder dynamics in patients with congenital neurological disease of the lower urinary tract. Bladder and native kidney anatomy and function must be considered prior to transplant in patients with declining GFR and predicted need for renal replacement therapy.

References

1. Danforth TL, Ginsberg DA. Neurogenic lower urinary tract dysfunction: how, when, and with which patients do we use urodynamics? Urol Clin North Am. 2014;41:445–52. ix.
2. Hellstrom WJ, Edwards MS, Kogan BA. Urological aspects of the tethered cord syndrome. J Urol. 1986;135:317–20.
3. Yener S, Thomas DT, Hicdonmez T, Dagcinar A, Bayri Y, Kaynak A, Dagli TE, Tugtepe H. The effect of untethering on urologic symptoms and urodynamic parameters in children with primary tethered cord syndrome. Urology. 2015;85:221–6.
4. Wein A, Dmochowski R. Neuromuscular dysfunction of the lower urinary tract. In: Campbell-Walsh urol. 10th ed. Philadelphia: Elsevier; 2012. p. 1909–46.
5. Wyndaele JJ. Correlation between clinical neurological data and urodynamic function in spinal cord injured patients. Spinal Cord. 1997;35:213–16.
6. McGuire EJ, Woodside JR, Borden TA, Weiss RM. Prognostic value of urodynamic testing in myelodysplastic patients. J Urol. 2002;167:1049–53; discussion 1054.
7. Leal da Cruz M, Liguori R, Garrone G, Leslie B, Ottoni SL, Carvalheiro S, Moron AF, Ortiz V, Macedo A. Categorization of bladder dynamics and treatment after fetal myelomeningocele repair: first 50 cases prospectively assessed. J Urol. 2015;193:1808–12.
8. Adzick NS, Thom EA, Spong CY, et al. A randomized trial of prenatal versus postnatal repair of myelomeningocele. N Engl J Med. 2011;364:993–1004.
9. Atala A, Bauer SB, Dyro FM, Shefner J, Shillito J, Sathi S, Scott RM. Bladder functional changes resulting from lipomyelomeningocele repair. J Urol. 1992;148:592–4.
10. Vij S, Wadick K, Luzney P, Myers J, Poggio E, Hertz B, Wood H. Assessing renal function in adult myelomeningocele patients: correlation between volumetric and creatinine-based measurements. J Clin Nephrol Ren Care. 2016;2:003.

11. DeLair SM, Eandi J, White MJ, Nguyen T, Stone AR, Kurzrock EA. Renal cortical deterioration in children with spinal dysraphism: analysis of risk factors. J Spinal Cord Med. 2007;30 Suppl 1:S30–4.

12. De Kort LMO, Bower WF, Swithinbank LV, Marschall-Kehrel D, de Jong TPVM, Bauer SB. The management of adolescents with neurogenic urinary tract and bowel dysfunction. Neurourol Urodyn. 2012;31:1170–4.

Lower Urinary Tract Anomalies

Michael Ingber

14.1 Introduction

Urethral and bladder anomalies are found during evaluation for refractory voiding symptoms or recurrent urinary tract infections with negative cultures. Some of the conditions which we describe in this chapter include diverticula of the bladder and urethra and genitourinary fistula. Occasionally, when voiding symptoms present with these anomalies, urodynamics may be indicated in order to evaluate baseline voiding function. Such studies may guide the practitioner in performing concomitant outlet procedures or provide a baseline to better understand how to handle future voiding complaints.

14.2 Urethral Diverticula

Urethral diverticula represent a common diagnostic dilemma in the field of Female Pelvic Medicine and Reconstructive Surgery. Symptoms often mimic other conditions such as urinary tract infections, overactive bladder, and interstitial cystitis/bladder pain syndrome. Oftentimes, a diverticula can be diagnosed when urinary tract infection is suspected, yet cultures are negative. The three "Ds" of urethral diverticulum, dysuria, dyspareunia, and dribbling post-void, are found in a minority of patients [1]. Occasionally cystoscopic evaluation may demonstrate one or more ostia of a diverticula, but oftentimes, cystoscopy can be unremarkable. In such cases, a T2-weighted MRI of the pelvis can demonstrate high signal intensity around the urethra and remains the diagnostic modality of choice for this condition [2].

Surgical excision remains the standard of care. Typical repair includes multiple layer closure, with nonoverlapping suture lines [3]. In cases where additional support is needed, a tissue interposition graft may be added as an added layer of closure. Whether or not to perform a concomitant anti-incontinence procedure at the time of the repair remains controversial; the author's opinion is that diverticula repair should be performed and, once healed, the outlet reassessed [4]. Subsequently, anti-incontinence surgery can occur if necessary.

The decision to perform urodynamics may be affected by the patient's preoperative continence status and possible planning for concomitant sling or outlet procedure.

14.3 Case Study

14.3.1 Patient 1

14.3.1.1 History

A 42-year-old female presented with urinary urgency, frequency, slow stream, and dysuria throughout the past year. She had been treated for presumed urinary tract infection by her primary care physician; however, symptoms recurred. Three of the four cultures which were sent during these episodes were negative. She denied fevers, chills, nausea, or vomiting. She complained of stress urinary incontinence with coughing, sneezing, and physical activity, requiring four pads per day. She had insertional dyspareunia.

14.3.1.2 Physical Examination

Complete physical examination was performed in this patient. The general examination revealed a thin woman in no apparent distress. Cardiac evaluation demonstrated a normal rate, regular rhythm, with no murmurs. There was no lymphadenopathy in the neck, groin, or axillae. Neurological examination revealed that she was alert and oriented × 3, with cranial nerves II–XII grossly intact. Psychological evaluation demonstrated a cooperative woman, with no depression or anxiety.

Pelvic examination revealed a well-estrogenized vagina with good anterior, apical, and posterior support. The urethra was hypermobile with 30° of mobility. Upon Valsalva maneuver, significant urinary incontinence was visualized per urethra. Palpation of the urethra revealed a fullness in the midurethra, suspicious for urethral diverticulum.

14.3.1.3 Lab Work/Other Studies

Cystoscopic evaluation was performed which revealed an ostium at the midurethral level.

T2-weighted pelvic MRI confirmed the presence of a saddlebag urethral diverticulum surrounding the midurethra (Fig. 14.1).

14.3.1.4 UDS

Findings

The urodynamic tracing of this case is shown in Fig. 14.2. The filling cystometrogram shows normal bladder compliance, with scattered uninhibited bladder contractions diagnostic of detrusor overactivity. The patient had normal initial sensations; however, strong desire was at a low

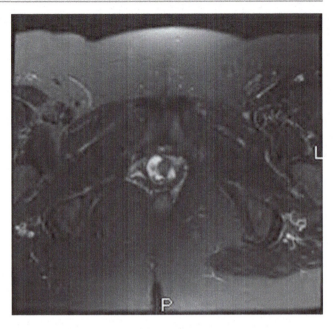

Fig. 14.1 MRI of the pelvis noting bright periurethral fluid-filled structure representing a midurethral diverticulum

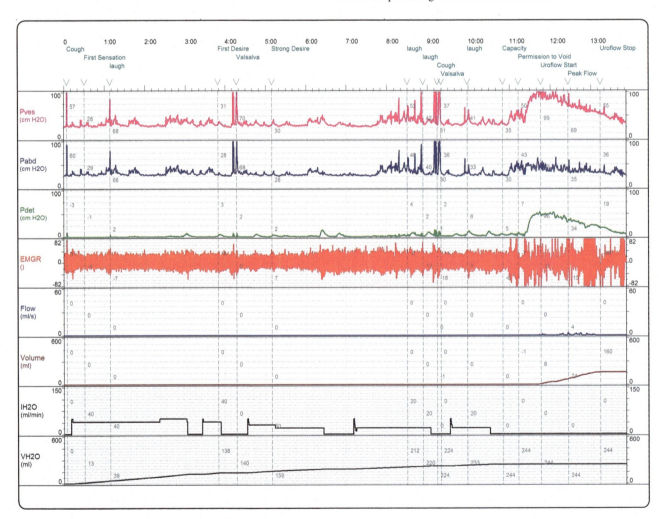

Fig. 14.2 Urodynamic study in a female with a urethral diverticulum

volume. Additionally, maximum cystometric capacity (MCC) was lower than the normal limits expected for this age at 160 mL. The voiding phase of the study demonstrated normal contractility, with elevated voiding pressures, with low urine flow.

In summary, it appears that this patient has detrusor overactivity which is likely secondary to a failure to empty based on outlet obstruction from the diverticulum.

14.3.1.5 Treatment Options

The standard of care for urethral diverticula is surgical excision, with multilayered closure. Consideration for tissue interposition must be given in cases where poor tissue quality hinders repair or in recurrent diverticulae.

Whether or not to address the outlet with respect to anti-incontinence surgery at the time of repair remains controversial. This patient has clear stress incontinence due to urethral hypermobility. Some argue that concomitant autologous fascial sling at the time of diverticulectomy can treat stress incontinence at the time of repair [2]. Lee reported rates of stress urinary incontinence after urethral diverticula repair and found that 75 % of women with preoperative stress incontinence continued to have stress incontinence postoperatively. Additionally, of 15 patients who had no prior stress urinary incontinence, 5 (33 %) developed de novo stress urinary incontinence postoperatively [5]. Nevertheless, it is the author's preference to stage incontinence surgery until after formal repair is performed and confirmed. One reason for this is due to the risk of recurrence of the diverticulum and difficulty in performing secondary repair after anti-incontinence surgery [6]. Urodynamics can be performed several months after repair in order to evaluate any persistent or de novo incontinence. If stress incontinence continues to be a bother, a subsequent synthetic midurethral sling can be performed in an outpatient setting and would be less morbid than an autologous fascial sling.

14.3.1.6 Clinical Course

This patient underwent a vaginal repair, with multilayered closure. No additional adjuvant flap was required, as the patient had a good watertight closure. The patient had a Foley catheter which remained for 2 weeks, at which point, a voiding trial was performed. The patient was seen at 6 months postoperatively, where the symptoms of urinary urgency, frequency, and dysuria were resolved. Some stress urinary incontinence also remained upon Valsalva with a full bladder. While a synthetic suburethral sling was offered, the incontinence was mild in nature, and therefore the patient elected conservative therapy in the form of watchful waiting.

14.4 Bladder Diverticula

Bladder diverticula represent a diagnostic challenge. There are two types of bladder diverticula that are found: congenital and acquired. The former is typically found in boys, at the ureterovesical junction (Hutch diverticulum), and the incidence is approximately 1.7 % [7]. While some are congenital, others develop as a result of obstruction at the bladder outlet over time. For example, in men with benign prostatic hypertrophy, chronic obstruction and high voiding pressure over time may predispose to diverticulum development. Occasionally, these acquired diverticula can become large enough to hold more urine than the native bladder itself [8].

Similarly, women with primary bladder neck obstruction, or increased outlet resistance due to a tight urethral sling, for example, may result in elevated voiding pressures. Initially, high voiding pressures will result in diverticulum development. Over time, with increasing size of the diverticulum, the diverticulum may become the path of least resistance during the voiding phase, resulting in incomplete emptying of the bladder, infrequent voiding, or recurrent urinary tract infections due to urinary stasis.

14.5 Case Study

14.5.1 Patient 2

14.5.1.1 History

A 56-year-old male presented with a history of urinary urgency, frequency, and slow urinary stream for the last 10 years. He had been on alpha blocker therapy throughout the past 5 years with minimal relief; despite medical therapy, he has had several episodes of urinary retention requiring catheterization. Over the past 2 years, however, the urgency and frequency had lessened. However, he stated he had infrequent voiding and feeling of incomplete emptying and urinary hesitancy.

14.5.1.2 Physical Examination

A complete physical examination was performed in this patient. The general examination revealed an obese male in no apparent distress. Cardiac examination demonstrated a normal rate, regular rhythm, with no murmurs or gallups. There was no lymphadenopathy in the neck, groin, or axillae. Neurological examination revealed that he was alert and oriented × 3, with cranial nerves II–XII grossly intact. Psychological evaluation demonstrated a cooperative male, with no agitation, depression or anxiety.

Genitourinary examination that included digital rectal exam was remarkable for a 60-g prostate, with no nodules or tenderness. The patient had a circumcised phallus, with no Peyronie's plaques. Testes were descended bilaterally without nodules or tenderness.

14.5.1.3 Lab Work/Other Studies

Noninvasive uroflow was poor, with <150 mL voided, despite a catheterized PVR of 950 mL (Fig. 14.3). Cystoscopy was performed in the outpatient setting. Urethroscopy was unremarkable, with no evidence for urethral stricture. The prostatic urethra demonstrated severe bilobar hypertrophy with no obstructing median lobe. The bladder had severe trabeculation throughout, consistent with chronic obstruction. There were several scattered cellules and a small-mouthed, large diverticulum found on the right lateral wall.

14.5.1.4 UDS

The cystometrogram phase of this study demonstrated normal bladder compliance, with no uninhibited bladder contractions. There was no evidence for intrinsic sphincter deficiency. The patient's first sensation was at 70 mL. First desire was at 297 mL, with a strong desire at 584 mL. The patient's maximum cystometric capacity was 750 mL. After the diverticulum was filled, despite knowing the total maximum capacity was likely over 1 L, he reached maximum cystometric capacity at 750 mL (Fig. 14.4). The voiding phase revealed the inability to void, despite a detrusor maximum pressure reading of 25 cm H_2O.

In summary, this patient appears to have a very large capacity bladder, due to the large diverticulum which he has acquired. This patient likely had a significant obstruction prior to development of the diverticulum, and, over time, has

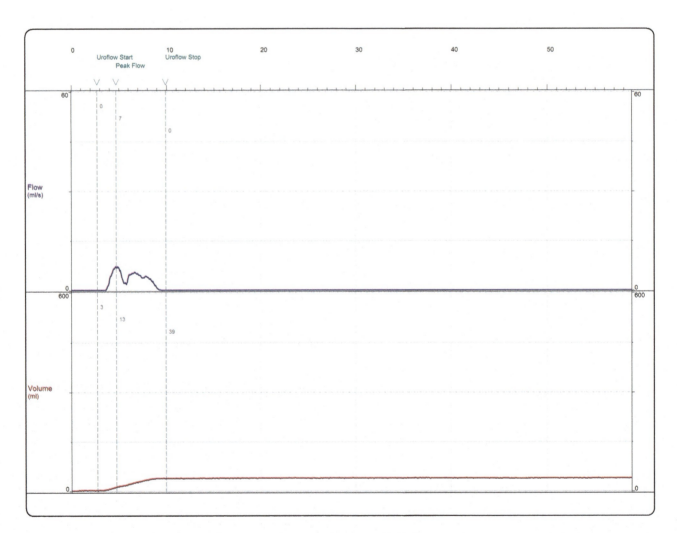

Fig. 14.3 Noninvasive uroflow, inadequate to determine proper flow given low voided volume

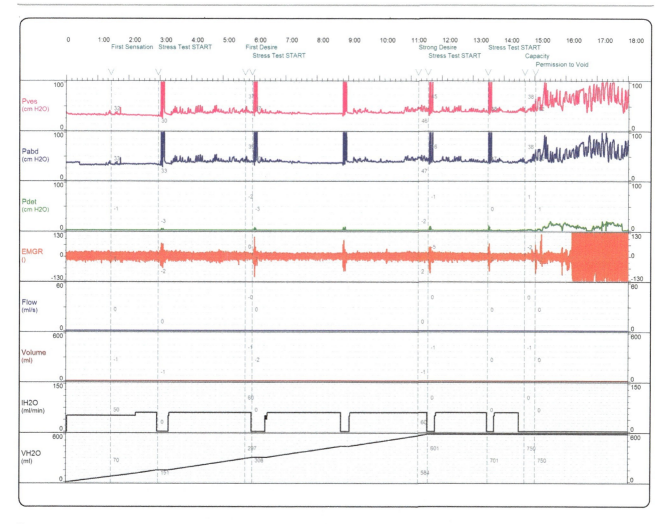

Fig. 14.4 Cystometrogram and pressure flow study in a patient with a bladder diverticulum

developed the diverticulum as a "pop-off" mechanism to relieve the obstruction. The urodynamic study demonstrates low detrusor voiding pressures, likely secondary to persistent filling of the diverticulum which was seen on videourodynamics.

14.5.1.5 Treatment Options

Bladder diverticula may be congenital or acquired later in life due to chronic bladder outlet obstruction. In men, this may be secondary to chronic benign prostatic hyperplasia. Over time, with chronic high-pressure voiding, diverticula can become essentially a "pop-off," as the path of least resistance. The diverticula by definition are non-muscle lined and can enlarge over time. In certain instances, it can become rather large, even having a larger capacity than the bladder itself. Incomplete emptying due to the diverticulum being a reservoir can lead to chronic retention symptoms, as well as infections or stones due to urinary stasis. In women, chronic obstruction leading to diverticulum development may be due to stricture disease, prior procedures which may increase outlet resistance such as midurethral slings, or prior urethral surgery. Fixing the diverticulum and relieving the outlet obstruction can treat the voiding dysfunction.

14.5.1.6 Clinical Course

This patient underwent a staged procedure, in order to both address his outlet obstruction as well as the large bladder diverticulum. A transurethral resection of the prostate was performed, and 1 month later, robotic-assisted laparoscopic diverticulectomy was performed. The patient tolerated the procedure well. Foley catheterization was performed for 14 days, at which point, a cystogram confirmed no evidence of leakage and a voiding trial was performed. The patient was able to void to completion, with a strong flow, and low postvoid residual. Additional follow-up at 3 and 6 months demonstrated persistent normal flow and low-volume post-void residuals.

14.6 Genitourinary Fistulae

A fistula is an abnormal communication between two structures. In female pelvic surgery, the most common fistulae encountered include vesicovaginal and urethrovaginal fistula. In developed countries, the most common type of fistula encountered is secondary to pelvic surgeries such as hysterectomy or procedures for urinary incontinence or pelvic reconstruction [9]. In developing countries, prolonged labor due to obstetrical obstruction can result in very large fistulae which present a major surgical challenge [10]. Cystoscopic evaluation and upper tract imaging, in order to rule out ureteral involvement in fistulae, are important factors in the diagnostic evaluation. Urodynamics have less of a role in preoperative planning; however, given the common lower urinary tract symptoms found both preoperatively and postoperatively, they can play a role in additional management.

14.7 Case Study

14.7.1 Patient 3

14.7.1.1 History
A 44-year-old female presented to the office with a history of severe stress urinary incontinence throughout the past 5 years. She complained of severe and insensate leakage, worse during the daytime, requiring six heavy pads per day. She had positional incontinence and severe urgency, mostly while active during the daytime.

Four years prior to presentation, she had a repair of a saddlebag midurethral diverticulum. The repair was done with a standard vaginal approach, utilizing a three-layer closure with nonoverlapping suture lines. No tissue interposition was done at the time. One year after repair, she was found to have a small urethrovaginal fistula, which was repaired in a similar fashion utilizing native tissue for repair providing a watertight closure.

14.7.1.2 Physical Examination
Physical examination was performed. The patient was well-nourished. Cardiac examination revealed a normal rate and rhythm, with no peripheral edema. The patient had normal respirations, with no chest wall tenderness. Abdominal examination was unremarkable for any masses or organomegaly. There was no tenderness to deep or light palpation. Neurological examination revealed that she was alert and oriented times three in no apparent distress. Psychological evaluation demonstrated she was cooperative and without depression or anxiety. Genitourinary examination demonstrated a well-estrogenized vaginal mucosa. There was no evidence for prolapse. She had marked incontinence per urethra upon Valsalva and cough. Urethral hypermobility of 45° was present. Pelvic floor squeeze strength was good.

14.7.1.3 Lab Work/Other Studies
Cystoscopic examination in the office was performed. The bladder was evaluated in its entirety and no evidence for papillary masses was seen. The ureters were visualized bilaterally with good efflux. Retroflexed view of the bladder neck was unremarkable. Urethroscopy demonstrated what appeared to be a residual diverticulum versus urethrovaginal fistula at the midurethra. With water flowing through the scope and the meatus occluded around the scope manually, it was evident that the irrigation fluid was leaking at the midurethral level, consistent with a recurrent urethrovaginal fistula.

14.7.1.4 UDS
Because of the patient's prior complicated urologic history, of both a urethral diverticulum repair and subsequent urethrovaginal fistula repair, urodynamic evaluation was performed to understand the patient's baseline detrusor and sphincter function (Fig. 14.5).

Cystometrogram demonstrated first sensation with uninhibited contractions at very low bladder volumes. Because of the low volumes producing discomfort, a stress test was done at lower volumes than usual. With 66 mL within the bladder, a Valsalva maneuver produced a significant detrusor contraction, resulting in leakage. With 170 mL in the bladder, the patient had reached capacity. A second stress test was performed at maximum cystometric capacity, and again, stress-induced urgency was visualized with another uninhibited detrusor contraction. Pressure flow was performed at a maximum cystometric capacity of 170 mL, during an involuntary detrusor contraction. Maximum flow was 7 mL/s.

In summary, this urodynamic study demonstrated stress-induced urgency. While the voiding phase appeared to produce a high detrusor pressure with slow flow, because the void was *involuntary*, we cannot conclude any obstruction in this case.

14.7.1.5 Treatment Options
This patient has a recurrent urethrovaginal fistula, along with stress-induced urgency, further complicating her stress urinary incontinence. Nevertheless, the dilemma of whether to address the urinary incontinence at the time of fistula repair exists. Some may offer addressing the stress urinary incontinence at the time of fistula repair with a concomitant biologic, autologous fascial, or even synthetic sling [11]. However, the author prefers to stage any incontinence procedures until after the fistula repair is complete.

In developed countries, urethrovaginal fistulae most commonly occur after previous vaginal surgery. Symptoms are variable as are techniques for repair. Because of the

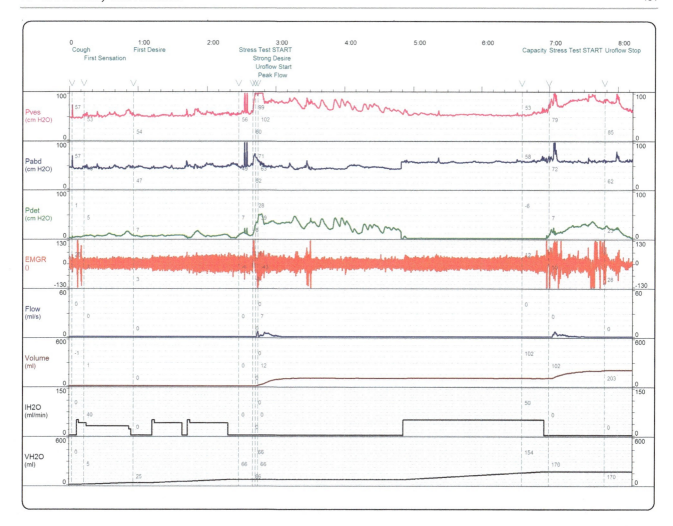

Fig. 14.5 Urodynamic evaluation of a patient with a urethrovaginal fistula, notable for stress-induced urgency

proximity of the urethral sphincter, patients with urethrovaginal fistula that occur within the proximal or midurethra are prone to de novo stress urinary incontinence after repair. In one study of patients undergoing urethrovaginal fistula repair, of 71 subjects undergoing repair, 37 (52.1%) developed stress incontinence after repair [12]. Some surgeons advocate the use of autologous fascia in order to correct stress incontinence during urethrovaginal fistula repair [13, 14], but the author typically prefers to wait until any fistula repair is complete. Once several months of healing has occurred, if the incontinence remains, it may be assessed, and a synthetic or autologous sling may be placed if necessary.

14.7.1.6 Clinical Course

This patient had a recurrent urethrovaginal fistula repair, with a multilayered closure. A Martius graft was utilized at the time of the repair given her recurrence. The patient's postoperative course was uneventful, with Foley catheter drainage for 14 days. A voiding cystourethrogram confirmed no evidence for obvious fistula. At 3 months postoperatively, the patient had marked improvement in her urinary leakage and no longer required any additional therapy.

14.8 Summary

Successful management of urethral and bladder anomalies is dependent on proper identification of the anomaly, understanding of the concomitant voiding dysfunction, and proper surgical repair. Urodynamics may be helpful in certain situations, when assessing preoperative voiding complaints or as a baseline prior to repair. When urodynamic parameters may alter the surgical repair, these studies should be performed.

References

1. Patel AK, Chapple CR. Female urethral diverticula. Curr Opin Urol. 2006;16(4):248–54.

2. Faerber GJ. Urethral diverticulectomy and pubovaginal sling for the simultaneous treatment of urethral diverticulum and intrinsic sphincter deficiency. Tech Urol. 1998;4(4):192–7.
3. Aspera AM, Rackley RR, Vasavada SP. Contemporary evaluation and management of the female urethral diverticulum. Urol Clin North Am. 2002;29(3):617–24.
4. Crescenze IM, Goldman HB. Female urethral diverticulum: current diagnosis and management. Curr Urol Rep. 2015;16(10):71.
5. Lee UJ, Goldman H, Moore C, Daneshgari F, Rackley RR, Vasavada SP. Rate of de novo stress urinary incontinence after urethal diverticulum repair. Urology. 2008;71(5):849–53.
6. Ingber MS, Firoozi F, Vasavada SP, Ching CB, Goldman HB, Moore CK, Rackley RR. Surgically corrected urethral diverticula: long-term voiding dysfunction and reoperation rates. Urology. 2011;77(1):65–9.
7. Powell CR, Kreder KJ. Treatment of bladder diverticula, impaired detrusor contractility, and low bladder compliance. Urol Clin North Am. 2009;36(4):511–25.
8. Tortorelli AP, Rosa F, Papa V, Alfieri S, Doglietto GB. Giant bladder diverticulum. Updates Surg. 2011;63(1):63–6.
9. LafayPillet M, Leonard F, Chopin N, et al. Incidence and risk factors of bladder injuries during laparoscopic hysterectomy indicated for benign uterine pathologies: a 14.5 years experience in a continuous series of 1501 procedures. Hum Reprod. 2009;24(4):842–9.
10. Muleta M. Obstetric fistula in developing countries, a review article. J Obstet Gynaecol Can. 2006;28(11):962–6.
11. Smith AL, Davila GW. Biologic grafted repair of urethrovaginal fistula and concomitant synthetic sling. Int Urogynecol J. 2013;24(5):729–30.
12. Pushkar DY, Dyakov VV, Kosko JW, Kasyan GR. Management of urethrovaginal fistulas. Eur Urol. 2006;50(5):1000–5.
13. Blaivas JG, Purohit RS. Post-traumatic female urethral reconstruction. Curr Urol Rep. 2008;9(5):397–404.
14. Golomb J, Leibovitch I, Mor Y, Nadu A, Ramon J. Fascial patch technique for repair of complicated urethrovaginal fistula. Urology. 2006;68(5):1115–18.

Index

A

AA. *See* Autoaugmentation (AA)
Abdominal leak point pressures (ALPPs)
    abdominal pressure, urethral meatus, 36
    defined, 13
    UDS, 81
AD. *See* Autonomic dysreflexia (AD)
American Urological Association (AUA)
    antibiotic prophylaxis, urodynamic studies, 6
    score, 56
Amyotrophic lateral sclerosis (ALS), 80
    Artificial urinary sphincter (AUS)
    AdVance™ transobturator sling, 46
    bladder outlet obstruction, 51
    description, 44
    postprostatectomy stress incontinence, 45
    surgical options, 44
    videourodynamics, 48
Augmentation cystoplasty (AC). *See also* Lower urinary tract dysfunction (LUTD)
    AA/ureterocystoplasty, 102
    bladder augmentation, 101
    BoNT-A, 103
    CIC, 102
    concomitant procedures, 102
    contracted tuberculous/bladder exstrophy, 102
    early complications, 103
    high-capacity, low-pressure reservoir, 101
    IC/BPS, 102
    indications, 102
    long-term complications, 103
    median bladder capacity, 102
    reservoir perforation, 103
    urodynamic studies, 103–106
    urologist's role, 101
AUS. *See* Artificial urethral sphincter (AUS)
Autoaugmentation (AA), 102
Autonomic dysreflexia (AD)
    bladder distension, 82
    constipation, 80
    defined, 28

B

Baden-Walker Grade 1 cystocele, 69
Benign prostatic hyperplasia (BPH)
    aging male population, 55
    AUA symptom score, 56
    benign prostatic enlargement, 55
    characteristic LUTS, 55
    DO, 56
    hyperplastic nodules, 55
    lab work, 57, 59, 60
    medical therapy, 56
    office-based surgical procedures, 56
    physical examination, 57, 58, 60
    PSA testing, 56
    risk factors, 55
    treatment, 58, 60, 62
    UDS, 57–62
Benign prostatic obstruction, 18
Bladder diverticula
    congenital and acquired, 127
    cystometrogram and pressure flow, 128, 129
    detrusor trabeculation with bilateral, 29
    diverticulum development, 127
    lab work, 128
    physical examination, 127–128
    and renal deterioration, 55
    treatment, 129
Bladder hypersensitivity, 22–24
Bladder infections, 89–90
Bladder neck obstruction. *See* Primary bladder neck obstruction (PNBO)
Bladder outlet obstruction (BOO). *See also* Benign prostatic hyperplasia (BPH)
    cystocele obstruction, 70–72
    demographic and urodynamic factors, 94
    diagnosis
        anatomic obstruction, 65–66
        functional obstruction, 66
    external sphincter, dysfunctional voiding, 72–73
    history and physical examination, 66
    iatrogenic
        bladder infections, 89–90
        stress urinary incontinence, 90–91
    lower urinary tract conditions, 94
    primary bladder neck obstruction, 67–69
    sling obstruction, 70
    symptoms in females, 65
    tracings, 73–78
    urodynamics, role, 66–67
    voiding dysfunction, 94
Botulinum neurotoxin A (BoNT-A) injections, 101, 103
BPH. *See* Benign prostatic hyperplasia (BPH)

C

Cerebrovascular accident (CVA), 80
Classic neurogenic bladder
    lab work, 111, 112
    physical examination, 111

Classic neurogenic bladder (*cont.*)
  small-capacity, overactive bladder, 110
  symptoms, 110
  tethered cord, 110
  treatment, 111
Clean intermittent catheterization (CIC)
  AA, 101
  artificial urinary sphincter, 115
  bladder emptying, 102
  high-grade reflux, female gender and initiation, 110
  intradetrusor injection, onabotulinumtoxinA, 30
  mucus production, 103
  myelomeningocele, 117
  surgical intervention, 58
  voiding diary, 104
CMG. *See* Cystometrogram (CMG)
Complex UDS systems
  electrodes, 2–4
  exam table, 4
  fluid media, 2
  fluoroscopy, 4
  intra-abdominal catheters, 2
  intravesical catheters, 2
  printing data vs. transmission to EMR, 4
  purchase and maintenance, 4–5
  software, 4
  uroflow meter, 4
  wireless systems, 4
Congenital neurogenic bladder, 123
Cough leak point pressure, 13
CVA. *See* Cerebrovascular accident (CVA)
Cystocele obstruction, 70–72
Cystometric capacity
  filling rate of bladder, 13, 58–60
  UDS, 13
  voiding diary, 12
Cystometrogram (CMG), 1, 28, 91, 95, 96, 98
Cystoscopy
  bladder wall trabeculation, 50
  "Christmas tree" appearance, 118
  evaluation, 126, 130
  normal urethra without strictures, 57
  obstruction/erosion/PBNO, 66

D
Detrusor contractility, 15, 44, 58, 62, 99
Detrusor external sphincter dyssynergia (DESD), 66, 67
  bladder trabeculation and diverticula, 30
  and dysfunctional voiding, 16, 17
  increased EMG activity, 29
Detrusor leak point pressure (DLPP)
  defined, 11
  upper tract deterioration, 11, 101
Detrusor overactivity (DO), 83, 86
  abdominal pressure, 35
  anticholinergics, 69
  bladder outlet obstruction with, 25
  compliance, 11
  continence postimplantation, 52
  defined, 12
  filling cystometry, 38
  history, 22
  idiopathic/neurogenic, 101–102
  labwork/other studies, 22
  patient with stress incontinence, 44
  phasic/terminal, 28, 32
  physical examination, 22
  stress-induced, 14, 15, 37–38
  terminal, 12, 13
  treatment options, 22
  UDS, 22
Detrusor pressure (P_{det}), 2
Detrusor sphincter dyssynergia (DSD)
  acontractile bladders, 102
  bladder phenotype, 116
  chronic obstruction, 83
  clinical history, 116
  description, 17
  dysfunctional voiding, 67
  fluoroscopy and UDS tracing, 76
  involuntary detrusor contraction, 86
  lab work, 116
  neurogenic obstruction, 80, 116
  physical examination, 116
  treatment, 116, 117
Detrusor underactivity, 16, 18, 28, 43, 72, 94
DLPP. *See* Detrusor leak point pressure (DLPP)
DO. *See* Detrusor overactivity (DO)
DSD. *See* Detrusor sphincter dyssynergia (DSD)

E
Electrodes, complex UDS systems, 2–4
Electromyography (EMG), 2, 3, 6, 16, 28, 29, 32, 45, 50, 66, 68, 72, 86
Electronic medical record (EMR), 4
  ethernet capability, 5
  printing data vs. transmission, 4

F
Federal Drug Administration (FDA), 29
Female SUI
  in abdominal pressure, 35
  complicated, 35, 36
  cystometry, 37–38
  de novo urinary storage symptoms, 39
  diagnosis of, 35
  DO, 35
  long-standing history, 39–41
  LPP, 36–37
  LUTS, 35
  mixed urinary incontinence, 35
  synthetic midurethral slings, 38–39
  UPP, 37
  urodynamics and surgical treatment, 35
Filling cystometry, 10, 37
Fluid media, complex UDS systems, 2
Fluoroscopy
  anatomy, urinary tract, 9
  bladder neck and external sphincter function, 66
  complex UDS systems, 4
  cystocele, 71, 72
  detrusor trabeculation with bilateral bladder, 29, 30
  Fowler's syndrome, 73
  radiology licenses, 4
  safety requirements, 4
  sling obstruction, 70
  structural anomalies, 28
  video-urodynamics, 2, 49
Fowler's syndrome
  dysfunctional voiding, 72–73

external sphincter relaxation, 66
history, 72–73
lab work/studies, 72
physical examination, 72
treatment options, 72–73
UDS, 72

G
Genitourinary fistula
cystoscopic evaluation and upper tract imaging, 130
lab work, 130
physical examination, 130
treatment, 130–131
UDS, 130, 131
vesicovaginal and urethrovaginal fistula, 130

H
Hinman-Allen syndrome, 66
Hypertension, 30–31, 45, 94, 116
Hypocontractility, 56, 79, 82
Hypothyroidism, 30–31, 85–87
Hypotonic/atonic bladder
lab work, 113–115
patients with myelomeningocele, 111
physical examination, 113
treatment, 115–116

I
Iatrogenic BOO
bladder infections, 89–90
SUI, 90–91
Incontinence quality of life questionnaire (I-QoL), 44
International consultation on incontinence questionnaire short form (ICIQ-SF), 44
International Continence Society (ICS), 2, 6, 21, 44, 78
InterStim® device, 29
Intra-abdominal pressure
mixed urinary incontinence, 35
rectal catheter placement, 83, 86
SUI, 43
Intravesical pressure, 2, 3, 7, 13, 29, 37, 45
Intrinsic sphincteric deficiency (ISD)
defined, 36
incontinence improvement, 38
MUCP values, 37
patients with ALPP/VLPP, 37
sling placement with leakage, 36
urethral hypermobility, 36
Involuntary detrusor contractions
associated urinary incontinence, 84
CMG, 28
DO, 12
I-QoL. *See* Incontinence quality of life questionnaire (I-QoL)

L
Leak point pressures (LPPs)
abdominal force evaluation, 36
defined, 37
leakage, radiographic visualization, 37
patient positioning, 37
urinary leakage, 37

Lower urinary tract dysfunction (LUTD)
augmentation cystoplasty, 101, 102
bladder symptoms, 101
characteristics, 101
clinical signs, 101
neurogenic, 104
pathophysiology, 101, 102
urologist's role, 101
Lower urinary tract symptoms (LUTS)
AUA, 56
POP, 93
UDS with prolapse reduction, 94
urinary urgency and diurnal urinary frequency, 45

M
Magnetic resonance imaging (MRI), 29, 83–85, 125, 126
Male SUI
24-h pad test, 44
AUS, 44
bulbourethral slings, 45
congenital and acquired neurogenic disorders, 43
cystourethroscopy, 44
Kegel exercises and penile clamp, 47, 48
LUTS, 45, 46
minimally invasive and nerve sparing approaches, 43
nonoperative interventions, 44
normal bladder cycling, 44
periurethral bulking agents, 45
postprostatectomy incontinence, 43
PVP, 50–52
quality of life information, 44
radical prostatectomy, 43
UDS, 44
urological practice and patient's quality of life, 43
Mixed urinary incontinence
filling cystometry, 37–38
intra-abdominal pressure, 35
patient's incontinence, 38
urodynamic evaluation, 36
VALUE trial, 38
Multichannel VUDS, 81, 83, 86
Multiple sclerosis (MS)
clinical patterns, 80
detrusor-external sphincter dyssynergia, 66
history, 83
labwork/studies, 83
neurogenic causes, obstruction, 66
physical examination, 83
treatment options, 83–85
UDS, 83
voiding dysfunction, neurogenic, 79–80
Myelomeningocele (MM), 80, 109–111, 113, 115, 116

N
Neurogenic bladder
CIC and anticholinergic medication, 110
classic (*see* Classic neurogenic bladder)
clinical evaluation, 110
description, 109
after fetal myelomeningocele repair, 109
micturition, 110
neuroanatomical pathways, 109
obstruction
hypothyroidism, 85–87

Neurogenic bladder (*cont.*)
    multiple sclerosis, 83–85
    quadriplegia, 80–83
  prenatal myelomeningocele repair, 109
  therapies, 109
  transplant evaluation, 116, 118–123
  urodynamic testing, 109
Neurogenic OAB
  hypertension and hypothyroidism, 30–32
  SCI, 29–31
Neurogenic voiding dysfunction, 79, 80

O
Obstructive voiding, 55, 79, 89, 90, 94, 101, 110
Occult stress urinary incontinence, 15, 22, 39, 94
Overactive bladder (OAB)
  bladder hypersensitivity, 23–24
  bladder outlet obstruction, 24–26
  DO, 22
  neurogenic (*see* Neurogenic OAB)

P
Parkinson's disease (PD)
  neurogenic OAB, 27
  urinary retention, 58
  urodynamic tracing, 31, 57
Pelvic organ prolapse (POP)
  BOO (*see* Bladder outlet obstruction (BOO))
  labwork, 95, 97
  with LUTS, 93
  middle-aged women, 93
  physical examination, 94–95, 97
  and SUI
    anti-incontinence procedure, 93
    CARE, 93
    concomitant colposuspension, 93
    MUS, 94
    urodynamic stress incontinence, 93
  treatment, 96, 98
  UDS, 95–98
Pelvic Organ Prolapse Quantification (POP-Q) system, 21, 95, 97
Percutaneous tibial nerve stimulation (PTNS), 22, 29
POP. *See* Pelvic organ prolapse (POP)
Post void residual (PVR), 17, 18, 21, 27, 44, 69, 109, 111, 116
Pressure flow studies (PFS), 28, 29
Pressure-flow urodynamic (PFUD) study, 9, 10
Primary bladder neck obstruction (PNBO), 19, 66–69, 75
Primary-progressive pattern, 80
Progressive-relapsing pattern, 80
PTNS. *See* Percutaneous tibial nerve stimulation (PTNS)
PVR. *See* Post void residual (PVR)

Q
Quadriplegia, 80–83

R
Relapsing-remitting pattern, 80
Renal transplantation, 102, 110, 123

S
Sacral neuromodulation (SNM), 29
Secondary progressive pattern, 80

Self-intermittent catheterization (SIC), 88
Sensory urgency, 28
Simple UDS systems, 1–2
Skene's duct cyst, 66
Sling obstruction, 69, 70, 89–91
Society of Urodynamics, Female Pelvic Medicine, and Urogenital Reconstruction (SUFU), 27
Spinal cord injury (SCI), 27–31, 80, 85
Stress urinary incontinence (SUI)
  female (*see* Female SUI)
  history, 90
  male (*see* Male SUI)
  physical examination, 90–91
  treatment options, 91
  UDS, 91 (*see also* Urodynamics)
Stress-induced detrusor overactivity, 14, 35, 37–38
SUFU. *See* Society of Urodynamics, Female Pelvic Medicine, and Urogenital Reconstruction (SUFU)

T
Three-way stopcock approach, 6, 7
Transurethral resection of prostate (TURP), 44, 51, 58

U
UPP. *See* Urethral pressure profile (UPP)
Urethral diverticula, 66
  cystoscopic evaluation, 125
  physical examination, 125–126
  symptoms, 125
  treatment, 127
  typical repair, 125
  UDS, 126–127
Urethral hypermobility, 36
Urethral pressure profile (UPP), 2, 4, 37
Urgency urinary incontinence (UUI), 22, 27, 28, 30, 94
Urgent PC® device, 29
Urinary incontinence, stress, 90–91
Urinary tract infection (UTI)
  gross hematuria, 85
  mucus production, 103
  nocturnal enuresis, 116
Urinary urgency, 21, 22, 32, 35, 38, 45, 47, 83, 89, 125, 127
Urodynamics (UDS)
  anticholinergics, 39
  ASC, 93
  benefits, 1
  bladder outlet, 36
  clinical obstruction, 17–19
  closure pressures, 36
  coarse sensation, 10–11
  complex UDS systems, 2–5
  compliance, 11–12
  concomitant anti-incontinence surgery, 94
  continence, 13–15
  contributory factors, 36
  contractility, 15–16
  contractions (detrusor overactivity), 12–14
  coordination, 16–17
  coarse sensation, 10–11
  cystometry, 12–13, 37
  detrusor function, 39
  diagnostic tool, 36
  incontinence, 9, 12, 14, 15
  ISD, 36
  LPPs (*see* Leak point pressures (LPPs))

midurethral sling, 18
mixed urinary incontinence, 38
multichannel, 3
occult stress incontinence, 94
POP and LUTS, 93
repetitive pelvic stress, 36
setup, 5–6
simple UDS systems, 1–2
synthetic midurethral slings, 38
troubleshooting, 6–7
UPP, 37
urethral hypermobility, 36
Urodynamics tracing, 90, 91
Uroflow meter, complex UDS systems, 4
UTI. *See* Urinary tract infection (UTI)
UUI. *See* Urgency urinary incontinence (UUI)

V
Valsalva leak point pressure (VLPP), 13, 37, 38, 44, 94
Vesicoureteral reflux (VUR), 80–83, 86–88
Videourodynamics (VUDS), 48, 49, 81, 83, 86, 87, 103, 111, 113, 116, 122, 129
Voiding cystourethrogram (VCUG), 11, 87, 120

W
Wireless systems, complex UDS systems, 4

Z
Zero pressure, 6